CW00473391

COMPLETE

BLOOD SUGAR
DIARY

WITH

DIABETIC LOG & FOOD JOURNAL

Phone No : _____

Email   : _____

Address   : _____

_____

_____

Date : _____

© PISTACHIO PUBLISHING

Personal Information & Medical Contacts

Personal Information

Name   : _____
Gender   : _____
Date of Birth : _____
Blood Group   : _____

Emergency Contact Details

Name   : _____
Phone No   : _____
Relationship : _____
_____

Doctor Information

Name   : _____
Phone No : _____
Notes   : _____
_____
_____

Pharmacy Details

Name   : _____
Phone No : _____
Address : _____
_____
_____

Additional Notes

_____
_____
_____
_____
_____
_____
_____
_____

Thank you very much for purchasing this book.

If you find the book helpful, consider leaving a **Review at Amazon.**

Your valuable feedback will help others and encourage us to create more quality products.

© PISTACHIO PUBLISHING

*All Rights Reserved. No part of this publication may be reproduced, sell, stored in a retrieval system, stored in a database and / or published in any form or by any means.

Content of the Book

Doctor Visits & Appointments - *Page 5-6*

Record doctor appointment details of each visit - instructions, medications, medical notes etc.

Medication Organizer - *Page 7-8*

This section can be used to record medication details & changes - oral agents, insulin, supplements etc. with dosages and instructions.

Tests, Labs & Check-ups - *Page 9*

This versatile section can be used to keep track of periodic labs, tests and health checkups - e.g FBS, HBA1C, BMI value, Cholesterol etc.

Daily Food & Blood Sugar Log - *Page 11-132*

This section has dedicated pages for each day to comprehensively track daily blood sugar levels, food, nutrition, activities, exercise, medication/insulin, blood pressure levels & more.

Accommodates for 122 days (full 4 months if used daily)

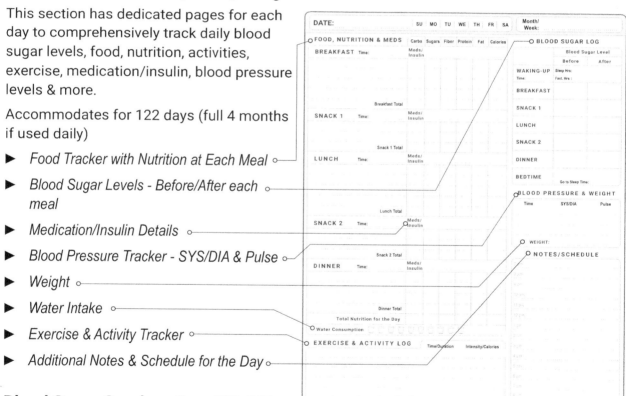

▶ *Food Tracker with Nutrition at Each Meal*

▶ *Blood Sugar Levels - Before/After each meal*

▶ *Medication/Insulin Details*

▶ *Blood Pressure Tracker - SYS/DIA & Pulse*

▶ *Weight*

▶ *Water Intake*

▶ *Exercise & Activity Tracker*

▶ *Additional Notes & Schedule for the Day*

Blood Sugar Graphs - *Page 133-136*

This helps to plot your daily blood sugar readings and visually compare them over the time.

Medical Notes - *Page 10 & 137-140*

Extra blank pages to record miscellaneous medical notes.

Blood Sugar Reference Charts

Fasting Blood Sugar/Plasma Glucose(FBS/FPG)

This test checks the fasting blood sugar levels. Fasting means after not having anything to eat or drink (except water) for at least 8 hours before the test.

Normal	3.9 to 5.4 mmol/L
Pre-Diabetes	5.5 to 6.9 mmol/L
Diabetes	7.0 or Above mmol/L

Two-hour Postprandial(After-meal) Test or Oral Glucose Tolerance Test (OGTT)

The OGTT is a two-hour test that checks the blood sugar levels before and two hours after drinking a liquid that contains glucose.

Two hours after a main meal test also should have similar values.

Normal	Below 7.8 mmol/L
Pre-Diabetes	7.8 to 11.0 mmol/L
Diabetes	11.1 or Above mmol/L

Random Blood Sugar (RBS)

Random blood sugar is measured at anytime of the day without having to fast first.

Normal value is **below 11.1 mmol/L**. Above **11.1** is considered Diabetes.

A1C / HBA1C

This test measures the average blood sugar for the past two to three months. It doesn't require to fast or drink anything.

Normal	Below 6.0
Pre-Diabetes	6.0% to 6.4%
Diabetes	6.5% or Above

Doctor Appointments/Visits

Date : .... Time : ....

Place: ....

Doctor : ....

Reason : ....

....

Notes : ....

....

....

....

....

....

....

....

Next Visit : ....

Date : .... Time : ....

Place: ....

Doctor : ....

Reason : ....

....

Notes : ....

....

....

....

....

....

....

....

Next Visit : ....

Date : .... Time : ....

Place: ....

Doctor : ....

Reason : ....

....

Notes : ....

....

....

....

....

....

....

....

Next Visit : ....

Date : .... Time : ....

Place: ....

Doctor : ....

Reason : ....

....

Notes : ....

....

....

....

....

....

....

....

Next Visit : ....

Doctor Appointments/Visits

Date : .... Time : ....

Place: ....

Doctor : ....

Reason : ....
....

Notes : ....
....
....
....
....
....
....

Next Visit : ....

Date : .... Time : ....

Place: ....

Doctor : ....

Reason : ....
....

Notes : ....
....
....
....
....
....
....

Next Visit : ....

Date : .... Time : ....

Place: ....

Doctor : ....

Reason : ....
....

Notes : ....
....
....
....
....
....
....

Next Visit : ....

Date : .... Time : ....

Place: ....

Doctor : ....

Reason : ....
....

Notes : ....
....
....
....
....
....
....

Next Visit : ....

Medication Organizer

Date	Medication/Insulin/Supplement	Dosage/Description

Medication Organizer

Date	Medication/Insulin/Supplement	Dosage/Description

Tests, Labs & Checkups

FBS	Target: ....
Date	**Value**

A1C	Target: ....
Date	**Value**

BMI	Target: ....
Date	**Value**

Date	Test	Values	Notes

Medical Notes

DATE:		SU	MO	TU	WE	TH	FR	SA	Month/ Week:

FOOD, NUTRITION & MEDS

	Carbs	Sugars	Fiber	Protein	Fat	Calories
BREAKFAST Time:	Meds/ Insulin					
Breakfast Total						
SNACK 1 Time:	Meds/ Insulin					
Snack 1 Total						
LUNCH Time:	Meds/ Insulin					
Lunch Total						
SNACK 2 Time:	Meds/ Insulin					
Snack 2 Total						
DINNER Time:	Meds/ Insulin					
Dinner Total						
Total Nutrition for the Day						

Water Consumption ⬜ ⬜ ⬜ ⬜ ⬜ ⬜ ⬜ ⬜ ⬜

EXERCISE & ACTIVITY LOG

	Time/Duration	Intensity/Calories

BLOOD SUGAR LOG

	Blood Sugar Level	
	Before	After
WAKING-UP Time:	Sleep Hrs: Fast. Hrs :	
BREAKFAST		
SNACK 1		
LUNCH		
SNACK 2		
DINNER		
BEDTIME	Go to Sleep Time:	

BLOOD PRESSURE & WEIGHT

Time	SYS/DIA	Pulse

WEIGHT:

NOTES/SCHEDULE

7 am
8 am
9 am
10 am
11 am
12 pm
1 pm
2 pm
3 pm
4 pm
5 pm
6 pm
7 pm
8 pm

Month/ Week: ....

FOOD, NUTRITION & MEDS

	Carbs	Sugars	Fiber	Protein	Fat	Calories
BREAKFAST Time:	Meds/ Insulin					
Breakfast Total						
SNACK 1 Time:	Meds/ Insulin					
Snack 1 Total						
LUNCH Time:	Meds/ Insulin					
Lunch Total						
SNACK 2 Time:	Meds/ Insulin					
Snack 2 Total						
DINNER Time:	Meds/ Insulin					
Dinner Total						
Total Nutrition for the Day						

Water Consumption

EXERCISE & ACTIVITY LOG

	Time/Duration	Intensity/Calories

BLOOD SUGAR LOG

	Blood Sugar Level	
	Before	After
WAKING-UP Time:	Sleep Hrs: Fast. Hrs :	
BREAKFAST		
SNACK 1		
LUNCH		
SNACK 2		
DINNER		
BEDTIME	Go to Sleep Time:	

BLOOD PRESSURE & WEIGHT

Time	SYS/DIA	Pulse

WEIGHT:

NOTES/SCHEDULE

7 am
8 am
9 am
10 am
11 am
12 pm
1 pm
2 pm
3 pm
4 pm
5 pm
6 pm
7 pm
8 pm

| DATE: | | SU | MO | TU | WE | TH | FR | SA | Month/Week: |

FOOD, NUTRITION & MEDS

	Carbs	Sugars	Fiber	Protein	Fat	Calories
BREAKFAST Time: _____ Meds/Insulin _____						
Breakfast Total						
SNACK 1 Time: _____ Meds/Insulin _____						
Snack 1 Total						
LUNCH Time: _____ Meds/Insulin _____						
Lunch Total						
SNACK 2 Time: _____ Meds/Insulin _____						
Snack 2 Total						
DINNER Time: _____ Meds/Insulin _____						
Dinner Total						
Total Nutrition for the Day						

Water Consumption ☐ ☐ ☐ ☐ ☐ ☐ ☐ ☐ _____

EXERCISE & ACTIVITY LOG

	Time/Duration	Intensity/Calories

BLOOD SUGAR LOG

	Blood Sugar Level	
	Before	After
WAKING-UP Time:	Sleep Hrs: Fast. Hrs :	
BREAKFAST		
SNACK 1		
LUNCH		
SNACK 2		
DINNER		
BEDTIME	Go to Sleep Time:	

BLOOD PRESSURE & WEIGHT

Time	SYS/DIA	Pulse

WEIGHT:

NOTES/SCHEDULE

7 am
8 am
9 am
10 am
11 am
12 pm
1 pm
2 pm
3 pm
4 pm
5 pm
6 pm
7 pm
8 pm

DATE:	SU	MO	TU	WE	TH	FR	SA	Month/Week:

FOOD, NUTRITION & MEDS

	Carbs	Sugars	Fiber	Protein	Fat	Calories
BREAKFAST Time: .... Meds/Insulin						
Breakfast Total						
SNACK 1 Time: .... Meds/Insulin						
Snack 1 Total						
LUNCH Time: .... Meds/Insulin						
Lunch Total						
SNACK 2 Time: .... Meds/Insulin						
Snack 2 Total						
DINNER Time: .... Meds/Insulin						
Dinner Total						
Total Nutrition for the Day						

Water Consumption ⊔ ⊔ ⊔ ⊔ ⊔ ⊔ ⊔ ⊔ ⊔ ⊔ ....

EXERCISE & ACTIVITY LOG

	Time/Duration	Intensity/Calories

BLOOD SUGAR LOG

	Blood Sugar Level	
	Before	After
WAKING-UP Time:	Sleep Hrs: Fast. Hrs :	
BREAKFAST		
SNACK 1		
LUNCH		
SNACK 2		
DINNER		
BEDTIME	Go to Sleep Time:	

BLOOD PRESSURE & WEIGHT

Time	SYS/DIA	Pulse

WEIGHT: ....

NOTES/SCHEDULE

7 am
8 am
9 am
10 am
11 am
12 pm
1 pm
2 pm
3 pm
4 pm
5 pm
6 pm
7 pm
8 pm

FOOD, NUTRITION & MEDS

	Carbs	Sugars	Fiber	Protein	Fat	Calories
BREAKFAST Time: .... Meds/Insulin						
Breakfast Total						
SNACK 1 Time: .... Meds/Insulin						
Snack 1 Total						
LUNCH Time: .... Meds/Insulin						
Lunch Total						
SNACK 2 Time: .... Meds/Insulin						
Snack 2 Total						
DINNER Time: .... Meds/Insulin						
Dinner Total						
Total Nutrition for the Day						

Water Consumption 🥛🥛🥛🥛🥛🥛🥛🥛🥛🥛

EXERCISE & ACTIVITY LOG

	Time/Duration	Intensity/Calories

BLOOD SUGAR LOG

	Blood Sugar Level	
	Before	After
WAKING-UP Time:	Sleep Hrs: .... Fast. Hrs :	
BREAKFAST		
SNACK 1		
LUNCH		
SNACK 2		
DINNER		
BEDTIME	Go to Sleep Time:	

BLOOD PRESSURE & WEIGHT

Time	SYS/DIA	Pulse

WEIGHT:

NOTES/SCHEDULE

7 am
8 am
9 am
10 am
11 am
12 pm
1 pm
2 pm
3 pm
4 pm
5 pm
6 pm
7 pm
8 pm

FOOD, NUTRITION & MEDS

	Carbs	Sugars	Fiber	Protein	Fat	Calories
BREAKFAST Time:	Meds/ Insulin					
Breakfast Total						
SNACK 1 Time:	Meds/ Insulin					
Snack 1 Total						
LUNCH Time:	Meds/ Insulin					
Lunch Total						
SNACK 2 Time:	Meds/ Insulin					
Snack 2 Total						
DINNER Time:	Meds/ Insulin					
Dinner Total						
Total Nutrition for the Day						

Water Consumption

EXERCISE & ACTIVITY LOG

	Time/Duration	Intensity/Calories

BLOOD SUGAR LOG

	Blood Sugar Level	
	Before	After
WAKING-UP Time:	Sleep Hrs: Fast. Hrs :	
BREAKFAST		
SNACK 1		
LUNCH		
SNACK 2		
DINNER		
BEDTIME	Go to Sleep Time:	

BLOOD PRESSURE & WEIGHT

Time	SYS/DIA	Pulse
WEIGHT:		

NOTES/SCHEDULE

7 am
8 am
9 am
10 am
11 am
12 pm
1 pm
2 pm
3 pm
4 pm
5 pm
6 pm
7 pm
8 pm

| DATE: | SU | MO | TU | WE | TH | FR | SA | Month/ Week: |

FOOD, NUTRITION & MEDS

	Carbs	Sugars	Fiber	Protein	Fat	Calories
BREAKFAST Time: .... Meds/ Insulin						
Breakfast Total						
SNACK 1 Time: .... Meds/ Insulin						
Snack 1 Total						
LUNCH Time: .... Meds/ Insulin						
Lunch Total						
SNACK 2 Time: .... Meds/ Insulin						
Snack 2 Total						
DINNER Time: .... Meds/ Insulin						
Dinner Total						
Total Nutrition for the Day						

Water Consumption 🥛🥛🥛🥛🥛🥛🥛🥛🥛🥛

EXERCISE & ACTIVITY LOG

	Time/Duration	Intensity/Calories

BLOOD SUGAR LOG

	Blood Sugar Level	
	Before	After
WAKING-UP Time:	Sleep Hrs: Fast. Hrs :	
BREAKFAST		
SNACK 1		
LUNCH		
SNACK 2		
DINNER		
BEDTIME	Go to Sleep Time:	

BLOOD PRESSURE & WEIGHT

Time	SYS/DIA	Pulse
WEIGHT:		

NOTES/SCHEDULE

7 am
8 am
9 am
10 am
11 am
12 pm
1 pm
2 pm
3 pm
4 pm
5 pm
6 pm
7 pm
8 pm

DATE:		SU	MO	TU	WE	TH	FR	SA		Month/ Week:

FOOD, NUTRITION & MEDS

	Carbs	Sugars	Fiber	Protein	Fat	Calories
BREAKFAST Time: Meds/Insulin						
Breakfast Total						
SNACK 1 Time: Meds/Insulin						
Snack 1 Total						
LUNCH Time: Meds/Insulin						
Lunch Total						
SNACK 2 Time: Meds/Insulin						
Snack 2 Total						
DINNER Time: Meds/Insulin						
Dinner Total						
Total Nutrition for the Day						

Water Consumption

EXERCISE & ACTIVITY LOG

	Time/Duration	Intensity/Calories

BLOOD SUGAR LOG

	Blood Sugar Level	
	Before	After
WAKING-UP Time: Sleep Hrs: Fast. Hrs :		
BREAKFAST		
SNACK 1		
LUNCH		
SNACK 2		
DINNER		
BEDTIME Go to Sleep Time:		

BLOOD PRESSURE & WEIGHT

Time	SYS/DIA	Pulse
WEIGHT:		

NOTES/SCHEDULE

7 am
8 am
9 am
10 am
11 am
12 pm
1 pm
2 pm
3 pm
4 pm
5 pm
6 pm
7 pm
8 pm

DATE: .... | SU | MO | TU | WE | TH | FR | SA

Month/Week: ....

FOOD, NUTRITION & MEDS

	Carbs	Sugars	Fiber	Protein	Fat	Calories

BREAKFAST Time: .... Meds/Insulin ....

Breakfast Total

SNACK 1 Time: .... Meds/Insulin ....

Snack 1 Total

LUNCH Time: .... Meds/Insulin ....

Lunch Total

SNACK 2 Time: .... Meds/Insulin ....

Snack 2 Total

DINNER Time: .... Meds/Insulin ....

Dinner Total

Total Nutrition for the Day

Water Consumption 🥛🥛🥛🥛🥛🥛🥛🥛

EXERCISE & ACTIVITY LOG

	Time/Duration	Intensity/Calories

BLOOD SUGAR LOG

	Blood Sugar Level	
	Before	After
WAKING-UP Time:	Sleep Hrs: Fast. Hrs :	
BREAKFAST		
SNACK 1		
LUNCH		
SNACK 2		
DINNER		
BEDTIME	Go to Sleep Time:	

BLOOD PRESSURE & WEIGHT

Time	SYS/DIA	Pulse

WEIGHT:

NOTES/SCHEDULE

7 am
8 am
9 am
10 am
11 am
12 pm
1 pm
2 pm
3 pm
4 pm
5 pm
6 pm
7 pm
8 pm

FOOD, NUTRITION & MEDS

	Carbs	Sugars	Fiber	Protein	Fat	Calories

BREAKFAST   Time: Meds/Insulin

Breakfast Total						

SNACK 1   Time: Meds/Insulin

Snack 1 Total						

LUNCH   Time: Meds/Insulin

Lunch Total						

SNACK 2   Time: Meds/Insulin

Snack 2 Total						

DINNER   Time: Meds/Insulin

Dinner Total						
Total Nutrition for the Day						

Water Consumption ⬜ ⬜ ⬜ ⬜ ⬜ ⬜ ⬜ ⬜ ⬜ ⬜

EXERCISE & ACTIVITY LOG

	Time/Duration	Intensity/Calories

BLOOD SUGAR LOG

	Blood Sugar Level	
	Before	After
WAKING-UP Time:	Sleep Hrs: Fast. Hrs :	
BREAKFAST		
SNACK 1		
LUNCH		
SNACK 2		
DINNER		
BEDTIME	Go to Sleep Time:	

BLOOD PRESSURE & WEIGHT

Time	SYS/DIA	Pulse

WEIGHT:

NOTES/SCHEDULE

7 am
8 am
9 am
10 am
11 am
12 pm
1 pm
2 pm
3 pm
4 pm
5 pm
6 pm
7 pm
8 pm

FOOD, NUTRITION & MEDS

	Carbs	Sugars	Fiber	Protein	Fat	Calories
BREAKFAST Time: __ Meds/ Insulin						
Breakfast Total						
SNACK 1 Time: __ Meds/ Insulin						
Snack 1 Total						
LUNCH Time: __ Meds/ Insulin						
Lunch Total						
SNACK 2 Time: __ Meds/ Insulin						
Snack 2 Total						
DINNER Time: __ Meds/ Insulin						
Dinner Total						
Total Nutrition for the Day						

Water Consumption ⬜⬜⬜⬜⬜⬜⬜⬜⬜

BLOOD SUGAR LOG

	Blood Sugar Level	
	Before	After
WAKING-UP Time:	Sleep Hrs: __ Fast. Hrs:	
BREAKFAST		
SNACK 1		
LUNCH		
SNACK 2		
DINNER		
BEDTIME	Go to Sleep Time:	

BLOOD PRESSURE & WEIGHT

Time	SYS/DIA	Pulse
WEIGHT:		

NOTES/SCHEDULE

7 am
8 am
9 am
10 am
11 am
12 pm
1 pm
2 pm
3 pm
4 pm
5 pm
6 pm
7 pm
8 pm

EXERCISE & ACTIVITY LOG

	Time/Duration	Intensity/Calories

DATE:	SU	MO	TU	WE	TH	FR	SA	Month/ Week:

FOOD, NUTRITION & MEDS

	Carbs	Sugars	Fiber	Protein	Fat	Calories
BREAKFAST Time: .... Meds/ Insulin						
Breakfast Total						
SNACK 1 Time: .... Meds/ Insulin						
Snack 1 Total						
LUNCH Time: .... Meds/ Insulin						
Lunch Total						
SNACK 2 Time: .... Meds/ Insulin						
Snack 2 Total						
DINNER Time: .... Meds/ Insulin						
Dinner Total						
Total Nutrition for the Day						

Water Consumption 🥛 🥛 🥛 🥛 🥛 🥛 🥛 🥛 🥛 🥛 ....

EXERCISE & ACTIVITY LOG

	Time/Duration	Intensity/Calories

BLOOD SUGAR LOG

	Blood Sugar Level	
	Before	After
WAKING-UP Time:	Sleep Hrs: Fast. Hrs :	
BREAKFAST		
SNACK 1		
LUNCH		
SNACK 2		
DINNER		
BEDTIME	Go to Sleep Time:	

BLOOD PRESSURE & WEIGHT

Time	SYS/DIA	Pulse

WEIGHT: ....

NOTES/SCHEDULE

7 am
8 am
9 am
10 am
11 am
12 pm
1 pm
2 pm
3 pm
4 pm
5 pm
6 pm
7 pm
8 pm

DATE: .... | SU | MO | TU | WE | TH | FR | SA

Month/ Week: ....

FOOD, NUTRITION & MEDS

	Carbs	Sugars	Fiber	Protein	Fat	Calories
BREAKFAST Time: .... Meds/ Insulin						
Breakfast Total						
SNACK 1 Time: .... Meds/ Insulin						
Snack 1 Total						
LUNCH Time: .... Meds/ Insulin						
Lunch Total						
SNACK 2 Time: .... Meds/ Insulin						
Snack 2 Total						
DINNER Time: .... Meds/ Insulin						
Dinner Total						
Total Nutrition for the Day						

Water Consumption ☐ ☐ ☐ ☐ ☐ ☐ ☐ ☐

EXERCISE & ACTIVITY LOG

	Time/Duration	Intensity/Calories

BLOOD SUGAR LOG

	Blood Sugar Level	
	Before	After
WAKING-UP Time:	Sleep Hrs: Fast. Hrs :	
BREAKFAST		
SNACK 1		
LUNCH		
SNACK 2		
DINNER		
BEDTIME	Go to Sleep Time:	

BLOOD PRESSURE & WEIGHT

Time	SYS/DIA	Pulse

WEIGHT: ....

NOTES/SCHEDULE

7 am
8 am
9 am
10 am
11 am
12 pm
1 pm
2 pm
3 pm
4 pm
5 pm
6 pm
7 pm
8 pm

DATE:	SU	MO	TU	WE	TH	FR	SA		Month/ Week:

FOOD, NUTRITION & MEDS

	Carbs	Sugars	Fiber	Protein	Fat	Calories
BREAKFAST Time:	Meds/ Insulin					
Breakfast Total						
SNACK 1 Time:	Meds/ Insulin					
Snack 1 Total						
LUNCH Time:	Meds/ Insulin					
Lunch Total						
SNACK 2 Time:	Meds/ Insulin					
Snack 2 Total						
DINNER Time:	Meds/ Insulin					
Dinner Total						
Total Nutrition for the Day						

Water Consumption ▢ ▢ ▢ ▢ ▢ ▢ ▢ ▢ ▢ ▢ ....

EXERCISE & ACTIVITY LOG

	Time/Duration	Intensity/Calories

BLOOD SUGAR LOG

	Blood Sugar Level	
	Before	After
WAKING-UP Time:	Sleep Hrs: Fast. Hrs :	
BREAKFAST		
SNACK 1		
LUNCH		
SNACK 2		
DINNER		
BEDTIME	Go to Sleep Time:	

BLOOD PRESSURE & WEIGHT

Time	SYS/DIA	Pulse
WEIGHT:		

NOTES/SCHEDULE

7 am
8 am
9 am
10 am
11 am
12 pm
1 pm
2 pm
3 pm
4 pm
5 pm
6 pm
7 pm
8 pm

DATE:	SU	MO	TU	WE	TH	FR	SA	Month/ Week:

FOOD, NUTRITION & MEDS

	Carbs	Sugars	Fiber	Protein	Fat	Calories
BREAKFAST Time: Meds/Insulin						
Breakfast Total						
SNACK 1 Time: Meds/Insulin						
Snack 1 Total						
LUNCH Time: Meds/Insulin						
Lunch Total						
SNACK 2 Time: Meds/Insulin						
Snack 2 Total						
DINNER Time: Meds/Insulin						
Dinner Total						
Total Nutrition for the Day						

Water Consumption 🥛🥛🥛🥛🥛🥛🥛🥛🥛🥛

EXERCISE & ACTIVITY LOG

	Time/Duration	Intensity/Calories

BLOOD SUGAR LOG

	Blood Sugar Level	
	Before	After
WAKING-UP Time:	Sleep Hrs: Fast. Hrs :	
BREAKFAST		
SNACK 1		
LUNCH		
SNACK 2		
DINNER		
BEDTIME	Go to Sleep Time:	

BLOOD PRESSURE & WEIGHT

Time	SYS/DIA	Pulse

WEIGHT:

NOTES/SCHEDULE

7 am
8 am
9 am
10 am
11 am
12 pm
1 pm
2 pm
3 pm
4 pm
5 pm
6 pm
7 pm
8 pm

DATE:	SU	MO	TU	WE	TH	FR	SA	Month/ Week:

FOOD, NUTRITION & MEDS

	Carbs	Sugars	Fiber	Protein	Fat	Calories
BREAKFAST Time:	Meds/ Insulin					
Breakfast Total						
SNACK 1 Time:	Meds/ Insulin					
Snack 1 Total						
LUNCH Time:	Meds/ Insulin					
Lunch Total						
SNACK 2 Time:	Meds/ Insulin					
Snack 2 Total						
DINNER Time:	Meds/ Insulin					
Dinner Total						
Total Nutrition for the Day						

Water Consumption 🥛🥛🥛🥛🥛🥛🥛🥛🥛🥛 ....

EXERCISE & ACTIVITY LOG

	Time/Duration	Intensity/Calories

BLOOD SUGAR LOG

	Blood Sugar Level	
	Before	After
WAKING-UP Time:	Sleep Hrs: Fast. Hrs :	
BREAKFAST		
SNACK 1		
LUNCH		
SNACK 2		
DINNER		
BEDTIME	Go to Sleep Time:	

BLOOD PRESSURE & WEIGHT

Time	SYS/DIA	Pulse

WEIGHT: ....

NOTES/SCHEDULE

7 am
8 am
9 am
10 am
11 am
12 pm
1 pm
2 pm
3 pm
4 pm
5 pm
6 pm
7 pm
8 pm

DATE: .... | SU | MO | TU | WE | TH | FR | SA

Month/Week: ....

FOOD, NUTRITION & MEDS

	Carbs	Sugars	Fiber	Protein	Fat	Calories
BREAKFAST Time: .... Meds/Insulin						
Breakfast Total						
SNACK 1 Time: .... Meds/Insulin						
Snack 1 Total						
LUNCH Time: .... Meds/Insulin						
Lunch Total						
SNACK 2 Time: .... Meds/Insulin						
Snack 2 Total						
DINNER Time: .... Meds/Insulin						
Dinner Total						
Total Nutrition for the Day						

Water Consumption ▢ ▢ ▢ ▢ ▢ ▢ ▢ ▢

EXERCISE & ACTIVITY LOG

	Time/Duration	Intensity/Calories

BLOOD SUGAR LOG

	Blood Sugar Level	
	Before	After
WAKING-UP Time:	Sleep Hrs: Fast. Hrs :	
BREAKFAST		
SNACK 1		
LUNCH		
SNACK 2		
DINNER		
BEDTIME	Go to Sleep Time:	

BLOOD PRESSURE & WEIGHT

Time	SYS/DIA	Pulse

WEIGHT:

NOTES/SCHEDULE

7 am
8 am
9 am
10 am
11 am
12 pm
1 pm
2 pm
3 pm
4 pm
5 pm
6 pm
7 pm
8 pm

FOOD, NUTRITION & MEDS

	Carbs	Sugars	Fiber	Protein	Fat	Calories
BREAKFAST Time:	Meds/Insulin					
Breakfast Total						
SNACK 1 Time:	Meds/Insulin					
Snack 1 Total						
LUNCH Time:	Meds/Insulin					
Lunch Total						
SNACK 2 Time:	Meds/Insulin					
Snack 2 Total						
DINNER Time:	Meds/Insulin					
Dinner Total						
Total Nutrition for the Day						

Water Consumption 🥛🥛🥛🥛🥛🥛🥛🥛🥛🥛

EXERCISE & ACTIVITY LOG

	Time/Duration	Intensity/Calories

BLOOD SUGAR LOG

	Blood Sugar Level	
	Before	After
WAKING-UP Time:	Sleep Hrs:	
	Fast. Hrs :	
BREAKFAST		
SNACK 1		
LUNCH		
SNACK 2		
DINNER		
BEDTIME	Go to Sleep Time:	

BLOOD PRESSURE & WEIGHT

Time	SYS/DIA	Pulse
WEIGHT:		

NOTES/SCHEDULE

7 am
8 am
9 am
10 am
11 am
12 pm
1 pm
2 pm
3 pm
4 pm
5 pm
6 pm
7 pm
8 pm

| | SU | MO | TU | WE | TH | FR | SA |

Month/ Week:

FOOD, NUTRITION & MEDS

	Carbs	Sugars	Fiber	Protein	Fat	Calories
BREAKFAST Time: Meds/ Insulin						
Breakfast Total						
SNACK 1 Time: Meds/ Insulin						
Snack 1 Total						
LUNCH Time: Meds/ Insulin						
Lunch Total						
SNACK 2 Time: Meds/ Insulin						
Snack 2 Total						
DINNER Time: Meds/ Insulin						
Dinner Total						
Total Nutrition for the Day						

Water Consumption ☐ ☐ ☐ ☐ ☐ ☐ ☐ ☐ ☐ ☐

EXERCISE & ACTIVITY LOG

	Time/Duration	Intensity/Calories

BLOOD SUGAR LOG

	Blood Sugar Level	
	Before	After
WAKING-UP Time:	Sleep Hrs: Fast. Hrs :	
BREAKFAST		
SNACK 1		
LUNCH		
SNACK 2		
DINNER		
BEDTIME	Go to Sleep Time:	

BLOOD PRESSURE & WEIGHT

Time	SYS/DIA	Pulse

WEIGHT:

NOTES/SCHEDULE

7 am
8 am
9 am
10 am
11 am
12 pm
1 pm
2 pm
3 pm
4 pm
5 pm
6 pm
7 pm
8 pm

FOOD, NUTRITION & MEDS

	Carbs	Sugars	Fiber	Protein	Fat	Calories
BREAKFAST Time: .... Meds/ Insulin						
Breakfast Total						
SNACK 1 Time: .... Meds/ Insulin						
Snack 1 Total						
LUNCH Time: .... Meds/ Insulin						
Lunch Total						
SNACK 2 Time: .... Meds/ Insulin						
Snack 2 Total						
DINNER Time: .... Meds/ Insulin						
Dinner Total						
Total Nutrition for the Day						

Water Consumption 🥛 🥛 🥛 🥛 🥛 🥛 🥛 🥛 🥛

EXERCISE & ACTIVITY LOG

	Time/Duration	Intensity/Calories

BLOOD SUGAR LOG

	Blood Sugar Level	
	Before	After
WAKING-UP Time:	Sleep Hrs: .... Fast. Hrs :	
BREAKFAST		
SNACK 1		
LUNCH		
SNACK 2		
DINNER		
BEDTIME	Go to Sleep Time:	

BLOOD PRESSURE & WEIGHT

Time	SYS/DIA	Pulse
WEIGHT:		

NOTES/SCHEDULE

7 am
8 am
9 am
10 am
11 am
12 pm
1 pm
2 pm
3 pm
4 pm
5 pm
6 pm
7 pm
8 pm

DATE:	SU	MO	TU	WE	TH	FR	SA	Month/ Week:

FOOD, NUTRITION & MEDS

	Carbs	Sugars	Fiber	Protein	Fat	Calories
BREAKFAST Time:	Meds/ Insulin					
Breakfast Total						
SNACK 1 Time:	Meds/ Insulin					
Snack 1 Total						
LUNCH Time:	Meds/ Insulin					
Lunch Total						
SNACK 2 Time:	Meds/ Insulin					
Snack 2 Total						
DINNER Time:	Meds/ Insulin					
Dinner Total						
Total Nutrition for the Day						

Water Consumption ▯ ▯ ▯ ▯ ▯ ▯ ▯ ▯ ▯ ▯ ....

EXERCISE & ACTIVITY LOG

	Time/Duration	Intensity/Calories

BLOOD SUGAR LOG

	Blood Sugar Level	
	Before	After
WAKING-UP Time:	Sleep Hrs: Fast. Hrs :	
BREAKFAST		
SNACK 1		
LUNCH		
SNACK 2		
DINNER		
BEDTIME	Go to Sleep Time:	

BLOOD PRESSURE & WEIGHT

Time	SYS/DIA	Pulse

WEIGHT:

NOTES/SCHEDULE

7 am
8 am
9 am
10 am
11 am
12 pm
1 pm
2 pm
3 pm
4 pm
5 pm
6 pm
7 pm
8 pm

DATE:		SU	MO	TU	WE	TH	FR	SA	Month/ Week:

FOOD, NUTRITION & MEDS

	Carbs	Sugars	Fiber	Protein	Fat	Calories
BREAKFAST Time:	Meds/ Insulin					
Breakfast Total						
SNACK 1 Time:	Meds/ Insulin					
Snack 1 Total						
LUNCH Time:	Meds/ Insulin					
Lunch Total						
SNACK 2 Time:	Meds/ Insulin					
Snack 2 Total						
DINNER Time:	Meds/ Insulin					
Dinner Total						
Total Nutrition for the Day						

Water Consumption ⬜ ⬜ ⬜ ⬜ ⬜ ⬜ ⬜ ⬜ ⬜ ⬜ ....

EXERCISE & ACTIVITY LOG

	Time/Duration	Intensity/Calories

BLOOD SUGAR LOG

	Blood Sugar Level	
	Before	After
WAKING-UP Time:	Sleep Hrs: .... Fast. Hrs :	
BREAKFAST		
SNACK 1		
LUNCH		
SNACK 2		
DINNER		
BEDTIME	Go to Sleep Time:	

BLOOD PRESSURE & WEIGHT

Time	SYS/DIA	Pulse

WEIGHT: ....

NOTES/SCHEDULE

7 am
8 am
9 am
10 am
11 am
12 pm
1 pm
2 pm
3 pm
4 pm
5 pm
6 pm
7 pm
8 pm

DATE:	SU	MO	TU	WE	TH	FR	SA	Month/ Week:

FOOD, NUTRITION & MEDS

	Carbs	Sugars	Fiber	Protein	Fat	Calories
BREAKFAST Time: Meds/Insulin						
Breakfast Total						
SNACK 1 Time: Meds/Insulin						
Snack 1 Total						
LUNCH Time: Meds/Insulin						
Lunch Total						
SNACK 2 Time: Meds/Insulin						
Snack 2 Total						
DINNER Time: Meds/Insulin						
Dinner Total						
Total Nutrition for the Day						

Water Consumption ☐ ☐ ☐ ☐ ☐ ☐ ☐ ☐ ☐ ☐

EXERCISE & ACTIVITY LOG

	Time/Duration	Intensity/Calories

BLOOD SUGAR LOG

	Blood Sugar Level	
	Before	After
WAKING-UP Time:	Sleep Hrs: Fast. Hrs :	
BREAKFAST		
SNACK 1		
LUNCH		
SNACK 2		
DINNER		
BEDTIME	Go to Sleep Time:	

BLOOD PRESSURE & WEIGHT

Time	SYS/DIA	Pulse

WEIGHT:

NOTES/SCHEDULE

7 am
8 am
9 am
10 am
11 am
12 pm
1 pm
2 pm
3 pm
4 pm
5 pm
6 pm
7 pm
8 pm

DATE:		SU	MO	TU	WE	TH	FR	SA	Month/ Week:

FOOD, NUTRITION & MEDS

	Carbs	Sugars	Fiber	Protein	Fat	Calories
BREAKFAST Time:	Meds/ Insulin					
Breakfast Total						
SNACK 1 Time:	Meds/ Insulin					
Snack 1 Total						
LUNCH Time:	Meds/ Insulin					
Lunch Total						
SNACK 2 Time:	Meds/ Insulin					
Snack 2 Total						
DINNER Time:	Meds/ Insulin					
Dinner Total						
Total Nutrition for the Day						

Water Consumption 🥛🥛🥛🥛🥛🥛🥛🥛 ....

EXERCISE & ACTIVITY LOG

	Time/Duration	Intensity/Calories

BLOOD SUGAR LOG

	Blood Sugar Level	
	Before	After
WAKING-UP Time:	Sleep Hrs: Fast. Hrs :	
BREAKFAST		
SNACK 1		
LUNCH		
SNACK 2		
DINNER		
BEDTIME	Go to Sleep Time:	

BLOOD PRESSURE & WEIGHT

Time	SYS/DIA	Pulse

WEIGHT: ....

NOTES/SCHEDULE

7 am
8 am
9 am
10 am
11 am
12 pm
1 pm
2 pm
3 pm
4 pm
5 pm
6 pm
7 pm
8 pm

FOOD, NUTRITION & MEDS

	Carbs	Sugars	Fiber	Protein	Fat	Calories
BREAKFAST Time: Meds/Insulin						
Breakfast Total						
SNACK 1 Time: Meds/Insulin						
Snack 1 Total						
LUNCH Time: Meds/Insulin						
Lunch Total						
SNACK 2 Time: Meds/Insulin						
Snack 2 Total						
DINNER Time: Meds/Insulin						
Dinner Total						
Total Nutrition for the Day						

Water Consumption ⬜⬜⬜⬜⬜⬜⬜⬜⬜⬜

EXERCISE & ACTIVITY LOG

	Time/Duration	Intensity/Calories

BLOOD SUGAR LOG

	Blood Sugar Level	
	Before	After
WAKING-UP Time:	Sleep Hrs: Fast. Hrs :	
BREAKFAST		
SNACK 1		
LUNCH		
SNACK 2		
DINNER		
BEDTIME	Go to Sleep Time:	

BLOOD PRESSURE & WEIGHT

Time	SYS/DIA	Pulse

WEIGHT:

NOTES/SCHEDULE

7 am
8 am
9 am
10 am
11 am
12 pm
1 pm
2 pm
3 pm
4 pm
5 pm
6 pm
7 pm
8 pm

| DATE: | SU | MO | TU | WE | TH | FR | SA | Month/ Week: |

FOOD, NUTRITION & MEDS

	Carbs	Sugars	Fiber	Protein	Fat	Calories
BREAKFAST Time: .... Meds/ Insulin						
Breakfast Total						
SNACK 1 Time: .... Meds/ Insulin						
Snack 1 Total						
LUNCH Time: .... Meds/ Insulin						
Lunch Total						
SNACK 2 Time: .... Meds/ Insulin						
Snack 2 Total						
DINNER Time: .... Meds/ Insulin						
Dinner Total						
Total Nutrition for the Day						

Water Consumption 🥛🥛🥛🥛🥛🥛🥛🥛🥛🥛 ....

EXERCISE & ACTIVITY LOG

	Time/Duration	Intensity/Calories

BLOOD SUGAR LOG

	Blood Sugar Level	
	Before	**After**
WAKING-UP Time:	Sleep Hrs: .... Fast. Hrs :	
BREAKFAST		
SNACK 1		
LUNCH		
SNACK 2		
DINNER		
BEDTIME	Go to Sleep Time:	

BLOOD PRESSURE & WEIGHT

Time	SYS/DIA	Pulse
WEIGHT:		

NOTES/SCHEDULE

7 am
8 am
9 am
10 am
11 am
12 pm
1 pm
2 pm
3 pm
4 pm
5 pm
6 pm
7 pm
8 pm

DATE:	SU	MO	TU	WE	TH	FR	SA	Month/ Week:

FOOD, NUTRITION & MEDS

	Carbs	Sugars	Fiber	Protein	Fat	Calories
BREAKFAST Time: _____ Meds/ Insulin _____						
Breakfast Total						
SNACK 1 Time: _____ Meds/ Insulin _____						
Snack 1 Total						
LUNCH Time: _____ Meds/ Insulin _____						
Lunch Total						
SNACK 2 Time: _____ Meds/ Insulin _____						
Snack 2 Total						
DINNER Time: _____ Meds/ Insulin _____						
Dinner Total						
Total Nutrition for the Day						

Water Consumption ☐ ☐ ☐ ☐ ☐ ☐ ☐ ☐ ☐ ☐

EXERCISE & ACTIVITY LOG

	Time/Duration	Intensity/Calories

BLOOD SUGAR LOG

	Blood Sugar Level	
	Before	After
WAKING-UP Time:	Sleep Hrs: _____ Fast. Hrs : _____	
BREAKFAST		
SNACK 1		
LUNCH		
SNACK 2		
DINNER		
BEDTIME	Go to Sleep Time:	

BLOOD PRESSURE & WEIGHT

Time	SYS/DIA	Pulse

WEIGHT: _____

NOTES/SCHEDULE

7 am
8 am
9 am
10 am
11 am
12 pm
1 pm
2 pm
3 pm
4 pm
5 pm
6 pm
7 pm
8 pm

DATE: .... | SU | MO | TU | WE | TH | FR | SA | **Month/ Week:** ....

FOOD, NUTRITION & MEDS

	Carbs	Sugars	Fiber	Protein	Fat	Calories
BREAKFAST Time: .... Meds/ Insulin						
Breakfast Total						
SNACK 1 Time: .... Meds/ Insulin						
Snack 1 Total						
LUNCH Time: .... Meds/ Insulin						
Lunch Total						
SNACK 2 Time: .... Meds/ Insulin						
Snack 2 Total						
DINNER Time: .... Meds/ Insulin						
Dinner Total						
Total Nutrition for the Day						

Water Consumption ▯ ▯ ▯ ▯ ▯ ▯ ▯ ▯

EXERCISE & ACTIVITY LOG

	Time/Duration	Intensity/Calories

BLOOD SUGAR LOG

	Blood Sugar Level	
	Before	After
WAKING-UP Time:	Sleep Hrs: Fast. Hrs :	
BREAKFAST		
SNACK 1		
LUNCH		
SNACK 2		
DINNER		
BEDTIME	Go to Sleep Time:	

BLOOD PRESSURE & WEIGHT

Time	SYS/DIA	Pulse

WEIGHT: ....

NOTES/SCHEDULE

7 am
8 am
9 am
10 am
11 am
12 pm
1 pm
2 pm
3 pm
4 pm
5 pm
6 pm
7 pm
8 pm

DATE:	SU	MO	TU	WE	TH	FR	SA	Month/ Week: ....

FOOD, NUTRITION & MEDS

	Carbs	Sugars	Fiber	Protein	Fat	Calories
BREAKFAST Time: .... Meds/Insulin						
Breakfast Total						
SNACK 1 Time: .... Meds/Insulin						
Snack 1 Total						
LUNCH Time: .... Meds/Insulin						
Lunch Total						
SNACK 2 Time: .... Meds/Insulin						
Snack 2 Total						
DINNER Time: .... Meds/Insulin						
Dinner Total						
Total Nutrition for the Day						

Water Consumption ⬜⬜⬜⬜⬜⬜⬜⬜⬜

EXERCISE & ACTIVITY LOG

	Time/Duration	Intensity/Calories

BLOOD SUGAR LOG

	Blood Sugar Level	
	Before	After
WAKING-UP Time:	Sleep Hrs: Fast. Hrs :	
BREAKFAST		
SNACK 1		
LUNCH		
SNACK 2		
DINNER		
BEDTIME	Go to Sleep Time:	

BLOOD PRESSURE & WEIGHT

Time	SYS/DIA	Pulse

WEIGHT:

NOTES/SCHEDULE

7 am
8 am
9 am
10 am
11 am
12 pm
1 pm
2 pm
3 pm
4 pm
5 pm
6 pm
7 pm
8 pm

DATE:	SU	MO	TU	WE	TH	FR	SA	Month/ Week:

FOOD, NUTRITION & MEDS

	Carbs	Sugars	Fiber	Protein	Fat	Calories
BREAKFAST Time:	Meds/ Insulin					
Breakfast Total						
SNACK 1 Time:	Meds/ Insulin					
Snack 1 Total						
LUNCH Time:	Meds/ Insulin					
Lunch Total						
SNACK 2 Time:	Meds/ Insulin					
Snack 2 Total						
DINNER Time:	Meds/ Insulin					
Dinner Total						
Total Nutrition for the Day						

Water Consumption 🥛🥛🥛🥛🥛🥛🥛🥛🥛🥛 ....

EXERCISE & ACTIVITY LOG

	Time/Duration	Intensity/Calories

BLOOD SUGAR LOG

	Blood Sugar Level	
	Before	After
WAKING-UP Time:	Sleep Hrs: Fast. Hrs :	
BREAKFAST		
SNACK 1		
LUNCH		
SNACK 2		
DINNER		
BEDTIME	Go to Sleep Time:	

BLOOD PRESSURE & WEIGHT

Time	SYS/DIA	Pulse
WEIGHT:		

NOTES/SCHEDULE

7 am
8 am
9 am
10 am
11 am
12 pm
1 pm
2 pm
3 pm
4 pm
5 pm
6 pm
7 pm
8 pm

DATE: .... | SU | MO | TU | WE | TH | FR | SA | **Month/ Week:** ....

FOOD, NUTRITION & MEDS

	Carbs	Sugars	Fiber	Protein	Fat	Calories
BREAKFAST Time: ...	Meds/ Insulin					
Breakfast Total						
SNACK 1 Time: ...	Meds/ Insulin					
Snack 1 Total						
LUNCH Time: ...	Meds/ Insulin					
Lunch Total						
SNACK 2 Time: ...	Meds/ Insulin					
Snack 2 Total						
DINNER Time: ...	Meds/ Insulin					
Dinner Total						
Total Nutrition for the Day						

Water Consumption ⊔ ⊔ ⊔ ⊔ ⊔ ⊔ ⊔ ⊔ ....

EXERCISE & ACTIVITY LOG

	Time/Duration	Intensity/Calories

BLOOD SUGAR LOG

	Blood Sugar Level	
	Before	After
WAKING-UP Time:	Sleep Hrs: Fast. Hrs :	
BREAKFAST		
SNACK 1		
LUNCH		
SNACK 2		
DINNER		
BEDTIME	Go to Sleep Time:	

BLOOD PRESSURE & WEIGHT

Time	SYS/DIA	Pulse

WEIGHT:

NOTES/SCHEDULE

7 am
8 am
9 am
10 am
11 am
12 pm
1 pm
2 pm
3 pm
4 pm
5 pm
6 pm
7 pm
8 pm

DATE:	SU	MO	TU	WE	TH	FR	SA	Month/ Week:

FOOD, NUTRITION & MEDS

	Carbs	Sugars	Fiber	Protein	Fat	Calories
BREAKFAST Time:	Meds/ Insulin					
Breakfast Total						
SNACK 1 Time:	Meds/ Insulin					
Snack 1 Total						
LUNCH Time:	Meds/ Insulin					
Lunch Total						
SNACK 2 Time:	Meds/ Insulin					
Snack 2 Total						
DINNER Time:	Meds/ Insulin					
Dinner Total						
Total Nutrition for the Day						

Water Consumption

BLOOD SUGAR LOG

	Blood Sugar Level	
	Before	After
WAKING-UP Time:	Sleep Hrs: Fast. Hrs :	
BREAKFAST		
SNACK 1		
LUNCH		
SNACK 2		
DINNER		
BEDTIME	Go to Sleep Time:	

BLOOD PRESSURE & WEIGHT

Time	SYS/DIA	Pulse

WEIGHT:

NOTES/SCHEDULE

7 am
8 am
9 am
10 am
11 am
12 pm
1 pm
2 pm
3 pm
4 pm
5 pm
6 pm
7 pm
8 pm

EXERCISE & ACTIVITY LOG

	Time/Duration	Intensity/Calories

DATE:	SU	MO	TU	WE	TH	FR	SA	Month/ Week:

FOOD, NUTRITION & MEDS

	Carbs	Sugars	Fiber	Protein	Fat	Calories
BREAKFAST Time: _____ Meds/Insulin _____						
Breakfast Total						
SNACK 1 Time: _____ Meds/Insulin						
Snack 1 Total						
LUNCH Time: _____ Meds/Insulin _____						
Lunch Total						
SNACK 2 Time: _____ Meds/Insulin						
Snack 2 Total						
DINNER Time: _____ Meds/Insulin						
Dinner Total						
Total Nutrition for the Day						

Water Consumption ⬜ ⬜ ⬜ ⬜ ⬜ ⬜ ⬜ ⬜ ⬜

EXERCISE & ACTIVITY LOG

	Time/Duration	Intensity/Calories

BLOOD SUGAR LOG

	Blood Sugar Level	
	Before	After
WAKING-UP Time:	Sleep Hrs: Fast. Hrs :	
BREAKFAST		
SNACK 1		
LUNCH		
SNACK 2		
DINNER		
BEDTIME	Go to Sleep Time:	

BLOOD PRESSURE & WEIGHT

Time	SYS/DIA	Pulse

WEIGHT:

NOTES/SCHEDULE

7 am	
8 am	
9 am	
10 am	
11 am	
12 pm	
1 pm	
2 pm	
3 pm	
4 pm	
5 pm	
6 pm	
7 pm	
8 pm	

DATE: .... | SU | MO | TU | WE | TH | FR | SA | **Month/ Week:** ....

FOOD, NUTRITION & MEDS

	Carbs	Sugars	Fiber	Protein	Fat	Calories
BREAKFAST Time: .... Meds/Insulin						
Breakfast Total						
SNACK 1 Time: .... Meds/Insulin						
Snack 1 Total						
LUNCH Time: .... Meds/Insulin						
Lunch Total						
SNACK 2 Time: .... Meds/Insulin						
Snack 2 Total						
DINNER Time: .... Meds/Insulin						
Dinner Total						
Total Nutrition for the Day						

Water Consumption 🥛🥛🥛🥛🥛🥛🥛🥛🥛🥛 ....

EXERCISE & ACTIVITY LOG

	Time/Duration	Intensity/Calories

BLOOD SUGAR LOG

	Blood Sugar Level	
	Before	After
WAKING-UP Time:	Sleep Hrs: .... Fast. Hrs :	
BREAKFAST		
SNACK 1		
LUNCH		
SNACK 2		
DINNER		
BEDTIME	Go to Sleep Time:	

BLOOD PRESSURE & WEIGHT

Time	SYS/DIA	Pulse
WEIGHT:		

NOTES/SCHEDULE

7 am
8 am
9 am
10 am
11 am
12 pm
1 pm
2 pm
3 pm
4 pm
5 pm
6 pm
7 pm
8 pm

DATE:		SU	MO	TU	WE	TH	FR	SA		Month/ Week:

FOOD, NUTRITION & MEDS

	Carbs	Sugars	Fiber	Protein	Fat	Calories
BREAKFAST Time: _____ Meds/Insulin _____						
Breakfast Total						
SNACK 1 Time: _____ Meds/Insulin _____						
Snack 1 Total						
LUNCH Time: _____ Meds/Insulin _____						
Lunch Total						
SNACK 2 Time: _____ Meds/Insulin _____						
Snack 2 Total						
DINNER Time: _____ Meds/Insulin _____						
Dinner Total						
Total Nutrition for the Day						

Water Consumption ◻ ◻ ◻ ◻ ◻ ◻ ◻ ◻ ◻ ◻

EXERCISE & ACTIVITY LOG

	Time/Duration	Intensity/Calories

BLOOD SUGAR LOG

	Blood Sugar Level	
	Before	After
WAKING-UP Time:	Sleep Hrs: Fast. Hrs :	
BREAKFAST		
SNACK 1		
LUNCH		
SNACK 2		
DINNER		
BEDTIME	Go to Sleep Time:	

BLOOD PRESSURE & WEIGHT

Time	SYS/DIA	Pulse

WEIGHT: _____

NOTES/SCHEDULE

7 am
8 am
9 am
10 am
11 am
12 pm
1 pm
2 pm
3 pm
4 pm
5 pm
6 pm
7 pm
8 pm

DATE:	SU	MO	TU	WE	TH	FR	SA	Month/ Week:

FOOD, NUTRITION & MEDS

	Carbs	Sugars	Fiber	Protein	Fat	Calories
BREAKFAST Time:	Meds/ Insulin					
Breakfast Total						
SNACK 1 Time:	Meds/ Insulin					
Snack 1 Total						
LUNCH Time:	Meds/ Insulin					
Lunch Total						
SNACK 2 Time:	Meds/ Insulin					
Snack 2 Total						
DINNER Time:	Meds/ Insulin					
Dinner Total						
Total Nutrition for the Day						

Water Consumption ▢▢▢▢▢▢▢▢▢▢

EXERCISE & ACTIVITY LOG

	Time/Duration	Intensity/Calories

BLOOD SUGAR LOG

	Blood Sugar Level	
	Before	After
WAKING-UP Time:	Sleep Hrs: Fast. Hrs :	
BREAKFAST		
SNACK 1		
LUNCH		
SNACK 2		
DINNER		
BEDTIME	Go to Sleep Time:	

BLOOD PRESSURE & WEIGHT

Time	SYS/DIA	Pulse

WEIGHT:

NOTES/SCHEDULE

7 am
8 am
9 am
10 am
11 am
12 pm
1 pm
2 pm
3 pm
4 pm
5 pm
6 pm
7 pm
8 pm

DATE: ....

| SU | MO | TU | WE | TH | FR | SA |

Month/ Week: ....

FOOD, NUTRITION & MEDS

	Carbs	Sugars	Fiber	Protein	Fat	Calories
BREAKFAST Time: .... Meds/Insulin						
Breakfast Total						
SNACK 1 Time: .... Meds/Insulin						
Snack 1 Total						
LUNCH Time: .... Meds/Insulin						
Lunch Total						
SNACK 2 Time: .... Meds/Insulin						
Snack 2 Total						
DINNER Time: .... Meds/Insulin						
Dinner Total						
Total Nutrition for the Day						

Water Consumption ▢ ▢ ▢ ▢ ▢ ▢ ▢ ▢ ▢ ....

EXERCISE & ACTIVITY LOG

	Time/Duration	Intensity/Calories

BLOOD SUGAR LOG

	Blood Sugar Level	
	Before	**After**
WAKING-UP Time:	Sleep Hrs: Fast. Hrs :	
BREAKFAST		
SNACK 1		
LUNCH		
SNACK 2		
DINNER		
BEDTIME	Go to Sleep Time:	

BLOOD PRESSURE & WEIGHT

Time	SYS/DIA	Pulse

WEIGHT:

NOTES/SCHEDULE

7 am
8 am
9 am
10 am
11 am
12 pm
1 pm
2 pm
3 pm
4 pm
5 pm
6 pm
7 pm
8 pm

DATE:	SU	MO	TU	WE	TH	FR	SA	Month/ Week:

FOOD, NUTRITION & MEDS

	Carbs	Sugars	Fiber	Protein	Fat	Calories
BREAKFAST Time: .... Meds/Insulin						
Breakfast Total						
SNACK 1 Time: .... Meds/Insulin						
Snack 1 Total						
LUNCH Time: .... Meds/Insulin						
Lunch Total						
SNACK 2 Time: .... Meds/Insulin						
Snack 2 Total						
DINNER Time: .... Meds/Insulin						
Dinner Total						
Total Nutrition for the Day						

Water Consumption ☐ ☐ ☐ ☐ ☐ ☐ ☐ ☐ ☐ ☐ ....

EXERCISE & ACTIVITY LOG

	Time/Duration	Intensity/Calories

BLOOD SUGAR LOG

	Blood Sugar Level	
	Before	**After**
WAKING-UP Time:	Sleep Hrs: Fast. Hrs :	
BREAKFAST		
SNACK 1		
LUNCH		
SNACK 2		
DINNER		
BEDTIME	Go to Sleep Time:	

BLOOD PRESSURE & WEIGHT

Time	SYS/DIA	Pulse

WEIGHT: ....

NOTES/SCHEDULE

7 am
8 am
9 am
10 am
11 am
12 pm
1 pm
2 pm
3 pm
4 pm
5 pm
6 pm
7 pm
8 pm

DATE:		SU	MO	TU	WE	TH	FR	SA	Month/ Week:

FOOD, NUTRITION & MEDS

	Carbs	Sugars	Fiber	Protein	Fat	Calories

BREAKFAST   Time: Meds/ Insulin

Breakfast Total						

SNACK 1   Time: Meds/ Insulin

Snack 1 Total						

LUNCH   Time: Meds/ Insulin

Lunch Total						

SNACK 2   Time: Meds/ Insulin

Snack 2 Total						

DINNER   Time: Meds/ Insulin

Dinner Total						
Total Nutrition for the Day						

Water Consumption 🥛🥛🥛🥛 🥛🥛 🥛🥛🥛

EXERCISE & ACTIVITY LOG

	Time/Duration	Intensity/Calories

BLOOD SUGAR LOG

	Blood Sugar Level	
	Before	After
WAKING-UP Time:	Sleep Hrs:	
	Fast. Hrs :	
BREAKFAST		
SNACK 1		
LUNCH		
SNACK 2		
DINNER		
BEDTIME	Go to Sleep Time:	

BLOOD PRESSURE & WEIGHT

Time	SYS/DIA	Pulse
WEIGHT:		

NOTES/SCHEDULE

7 am
8 am
9 am
10 am
11 am
12 pm
1 pm
2 pm
3 pm
4 pm
5 pm
6 pm
7 pm
8 pm

FOOD, NUTRITION & MEDS

	Carbs	Sugars	Fiber	Protein	Fat	Calories
BREAKFAST Time: .... Meds/ Insulin						
Breakfast Total						
SNACK 1 Time: .... Meds/ Insulin						
Snack 1 Total						
LUNCH Time: .... Meds/ Insulin						
Lunch Total						
SNACK 2 Time: .... Meds/ Insulin						
Snack 2 Total						
DINNER Time: .... Meds/ Insulin						
Dinner Total						
Total Nutrition for the Day						

Water Consumption ▢ ▢ ▢ ▢ ▢ ▢ ▢ ▢ ▢ ▢ ....

EXERCISE & ACTIVITY LOG

	Time/Duration	Intensity/Calories

BLOOD SUGAR LOG

	Blood Sugar Level	
	Before	After
WAKING-UP Time:	Sleep Hrs: .... Fast. Hrs :	
BREAKFAST		
SNACK 1		
LUNCH		
SNACK 2		
DINNER		
BEDTIME	Go to Sleep Time:	

BLOOD PRESSURE & WEIGHT

Time	SYS/DIA	Pulse

WEIGHT: ....

NOTES/SCHEDULE

7 am
8 am
9 am
10 am
11 am
12 pm
1 pm
2 pm
3 pm
4 pm
5 pm
6 pm
7 pm
8 pm

DATE: .... SU | MO | TU | WE | TH | FR | SA

Month/ Week: ....

FOOD, NUTRITION & MEDS

	Carbs	Sugars	Fiber	Protein	Fat	Calories
BREAKFAST Time: .... Meds/Insulin						
Breakfast Total						
SNACK 1 Time: .... Meds/Insulin						
Snack 1 Total						
LUNCH Time: .... Meds/Insulin						
Lunch Total						
SNACK 2 Time: .... Meds/Insulin						
Snack 2 Total						
DINNER Time: .... Meds/Insulin						
Dinner Total						
Total Nutrition for the Day						

Water Consumption ⬜ ⬜ ⬜ ⬜ ⬜ ⬜ ⬜ ⬜ ⬜ ⬜

EXERCISE & ACTIVITY LOG

Time/Duration   Intensity/Calories

BLOOD SUGAR LOG

	Blood Sugar Level	
	Before	After
WAKING-UP Time:	Sleep Hrs: Fast. Hrs :	
BREAKFAST		
SNACK 1		
LUNCH		
SNACK 2		
DINNER		
BEDTIME	Go to Sleep Time:	

BLOOD PRESSURE & WEIGHT

Time	SYS/DIA	Pulse

WEIGHT:

NOTES/SCHEDULE

7 am
8 am
9 am
10 am
11 am
12 pm
1 pm
2 pm
3 pm
4 pm
5 pm
6 pm
7 pm
8 pm

DATE: .... | SU | MO | TU | WE | TH | FR | SA

Month/ Week: ....

FOOD, NUTRITION & MEDS

	Carbs	Sugars	Fiber	Protein	Fat	Calories
BREAKFAST Time: .... Meds/ Insulin						
Breakfast Total						
SNACK 1 Time: .... Meds/ Insulin						
Snack 1 Total						
LUNCH Time: .... Meds/ Insulin						
Lunch Total						
SNACK 2 Time: .... Meds/ Insulin						
Snack 2 Total						
DINNER Time: .... Meds/ Insulin						
Dinner Total						
Total Nutrition for the Day						

Water Consumption ⬦ ⬦ ⬦ ⬦ ⬦ ⬦ ⬦ ⬦ ⬦ ⬦

EXERCISE & ACTIVITY LOG

	Time/Duration	Intensity/Calories

BLOOD SUGAR LOG

	Blood Sugar Level	
	Before	After
WAKING-UP Time:	Sleep Hrs: Fast. Hrs :	
BREAKFAST		
SNACK 1		
LUNCH		
SNACK 2		
DINNER		
BEDTIME	Go to Sleep Time:	

BLOOD PRESSURE & WEIGHT

Time	SYS/DIA	Pulse

WEIGHT: ....

NOTES/SCHEDULE

7 am
8 am
9 am
10 am
11 am
12 pm
1 pm
2 pm
3 pm
4 pm
5 pm
6 pm
7 pm
8 pm

DATE:	SU	MO	TU	WE	TH	FR	SA	Month/ Week:

FOOD, NUTRITION & MEDS

	Carbs	Sugars	Fiber	Protein	Fat	Calories
BREAKFAST Time: — Meds/ Insulin						
Breakfast Total						
SNACK 1 Time: — Meds/ Insulin						
Snack 1 Total						
LUNCH Time: — Meds/ Insulin						
Lunch Total						
SNACK 2 Time: — Meds/ Insulin						
Snack 2 Total						
DINNER Time: — Meds/ Insulin						
Dinner Total						
Total Nutrition for the Day						

Water Consumption ⬚⬚⬚⬚ ⬚⬚⬚⬚ ⬚⬚

EXERCISE & ACTIVITY LOG

	Time/Duration	Intensity/Calories

BLOOD SUGAR LOG

	Blood Sugar Level	
	Before	After
WAKING-UP Time:	Sleep Hrs: Fast. Hrs :	
BREAKFAST		
SNACK 1		
LUNCH		
SNACK 2		
DINNER		
BEDTIME	Go to Sleep Time:	

BLOOD PRESSURE & WEIGHT

Time	SYS/DIA	Pulse

WEIGHT:

NOTES/SCHEDULE

7 am

8 am

9 am

10 am

11 am

12 pm

1 pm

2 pm

3 pm

4 pm

5 pm

6 pm

7 pm

8 pm

| | SU | MO | TU | WE | TH | FR | SA |

Month/Week:

FOOD, NUTRITION & MEDS

	Carbs	Sugars	Fiber	Protein	Fat	Calories
BREAKFAST Time: .... Meds/Insulin						
Breakfast Total						
SNACK 1 Time: .... Meds/Insulin						
Snack 1 Total						
LUNCH Time: .... Meds/Insulin						
Lunch Total						
SNACK 2 Time: .... Meds/Insulin						
Snack 2 Total						
DINNER Time: .... Meds/Insulin						
Dinner Total						
Total Nutrition for the Day						

Water Consumption ☐ ☐ ☐ ☐ ☐ ☐ ☐ ☐ ☐ ....

EXERCISE & ACTIVITY LOG

	Time/Duration	Intensity/Calories

BLOOD SUGAR LOG

	Blood Sugar Level	
	Before	After
WAKING-UP Time:	Sleep Hrs: Fast. Hrs :	
BREAKFAST		
SNACK 1		
LUNCH		
SNACK 2		
DINNER		
BEDTIME	Go to Sleep Time:	

BLOOD PRESSURE & WEIGHT

Time	SYS/DIA	Pulse

WEIGHT: ....

NOTES/SCHEDULE

7 am
8 am
9 am
10 am
11 am
12 pm
1 pm
2 pm
3 pm
4 pm
5 pm
6 pm
7 pm
8 pm

DATE: .... | SU | MO | TU | WE | TH | FR | SA

Month/ Week: ....

FOOD, NUTRITION & MEDS

	Carbs	Sugars	Fiber	Protein	Fat	Calories

BREAKFAST Time: ....

Meds/ Insulin ....

Breakfast Total

SNACK 1 Time: ....

Meds/ Insulin ....

Snack 1 Total

LUNCH Time: ....

Meds/ Insulin ....

Lunch Total

SNACK 2 Time: ....

Meds/ Insulin ....

Snack 2 Total

DINNER Time: ....

Meds/ Insulin ....

Dinner Total

Total Nutrition for the Day

Water Consumption

EXERCISE & ACTIVITY LOG

	Time/Duration	Intensity/Calories

BLOOD SUGAR LOG

	Blood Sugar Level	
	Before	After
WAKING-UP Time:	Sleep Hrs: ..... Fast. Hrs :	
BREAKFAST		
SNACK 1		
LUNCH		
SNACK 2		
DINNER		
BEDTIME	Go to Sleep Time:	

BLOOD PRESSURE & WEIGHT

Time	SYS/DIA	Pulse

WEIGHT: ....

NOTES/SCHEDULE

7 am
8 am
9 am
10 am
11 am
12 pm
1 pm
2 pm
3 pm
4 pm
5 pm
6 pm
7 pm
8 pm

DATE: .... | SU | MO | TU | WE | TH | FR | SA

Month/Week: ....

FOOD, NUTRITION & MEDS

	Carbs	Sugars	Fiber	Protein	Fat	Calories
BREAKFAST Time: .... Meds/Insulin						
Breakfast Total						
SNACK 1 Time: .... Meds/Insulin						
Snack 1 Total						
LUNCH Time: .... Meds/Insulin						
Lunch Total						
SNACK 2 Time: .... Meds/Insulin						
Snack 2 Total						
DINNER Time: .... Meds/Insulin						
Dinner Total						
Total Nutrition for the Day						

Water Consumption 🥛🥛🥛🥛🥛🥛🥛🥛🥛🥛 ....

EXERCISE & ACTIVITY LOG

	Time/Duration	Intensity/Calories

BLOOD SUGAR LOG

	Blood Sugar Level	
	Before	After
WAKING-UP Time:	Sleep Hrs: .... Fast. Hrs :	
BREAKFAST		
SNACK 1		
LUNCH		
SNACK 2		
DINNER		
BEDTIME	Go to Sleep Time:	

BLOOD PRESSURE & WEIGHT

Time	SYS/DIA	Pulse
WEIGHT:		

NOTES/SCHEDULE

7 am
8 am
9 am
10 am
11 am
12 pm
1 pm
2 pm
3 pm
4 pm
5 pm
6 pm
7 pm
8 pm

| SU | MO | TU | WE | TH | FR | SA |

Month/ Week:

FOOD, NUTRITION & MEDS

	Carbs	Sugars	Fiber	Protein	Fat	Calories

BREAKFAST   Time:

Meds/ Insulin

Breakfast Total						

SNACK 1   Time:

Meds/ Insulin

Snack 1 Total						

LUNCH   Time:

Meds/ Insulin

Lunch Total						

SNACK 2   Time:

Meds/ Insulin

Snack 2 Total						

DINNER   Time:

Meds/ Insulin

Dinner Total						
Total Nutrition for the Day						

Water Consumption

EXERCISE & ACTIVITY LOG

Time/Duration   Intensity/Calories

BLOOD SUGAR LOG

	Blood Sugar Level	
	Before	After
WAKING-UP Time:	Sleep Hrs: Fast. Hrs :	
BREAKFAST		
SNACK 1		
LUNCH		
SNACK 2		
DINNER		
BEDTIME	Go to Sleep Time:	

BLOOD PRESSURE & WEIGHT

Time	SYS/DIA	Pulse

WEIGHT:

NOTES/SCHEDULE

7 am
8 am
9 am
10 am
11 am
12 pm
1 pm
2 pm
3 pm
4 pm
5 pm
6 pm
7 pm
8 pm

| DATE: | SU | MO | TU | WE | TH | FR | SA | | Month/ Week: .... |

FOOD, NUTRITION & MEDS

	Carbs	Sugars	Fiber	Protein	Fat	Calories
BREAKFAST Time: .... Meds/ Insulin						
Breakfast Total						
SNACK 1 Time: .... Meds/ Insulin						
Snack 1 Total						
LUNCH Time: .... Meds/ Insulin						
Lunch Total						
SNACK 2 Time: .... Meds/ Insulin						
Snack 2 Total						
DINNER Time: .... Meds/ Insulin						
Dinner Total						
Total Nutrition for the Day						

Water Consumption ☐ ☐ ☐ ☐ ☐ ☐ ☐ ☐ ☐ ......

EXERCISE & ACTIVITY LOG

	Time/Duration	Intensity/Calories

BLOOD SUGAR LOG

	Blood Sugar Level	
	Before	After
WAKING-UP Time:	Sleep Hrs: Fast. Hrs :	
BREAKFAST		
SNACK 1		
LUNCH		
SNACK 2		
DINNER		
BEDTIME	Go to Sleep Time:	

BLOOD PRESSURE & WEIGHT

Time	SYS/DIA	Pulse
WEIGHT:		

NOTES/SCHEDULE

7 am
8 am
9 am
10 am
11 am
12 pm
1 pm
2 pm
3 pm
4 pm
5 pm
6 pm
7 pm
8 pm

DATE: .... | SU | MO | TU | WE | TH | FR | SA

Month/ Week: ....

FOOD, NUTRITION & MEDS

	Carbs	Sugars	Fiber	Protein	Fat	Calories
BREAKFAST Time: .... Meds/ Insulin						
Breakfast Total						
SNACK 1 Time: .... Meds/ Insulin						
Snack 1 Total						
LUNCH Time: .... Meds/ Insulin						
Lunch Total						
SNACK 2 Time: .... Meds/ Insulin						
Snack 2 Total						
DINNER Time: .... Meds/ Insulin						
Dinner Total						
Total Nutrition for the Day						

Water Consumption ☐ ☐ ☐ ☐ ☐ ☐ ☐ ☐ ☐ ....

EXERCISE & ACTIVITY LOG

	Time/Duration	Intensity/Calories

BLOOD SUGAR LOG

	Blood Sugar Level	
	Before	After
WAKING-UP Time:	Sleep Hrs: Fast. Hrs :	
BREAKFAST		
SNACK 1		
LUNCH		
SNACK 2		
DINNER		
BEDTIME	Go to Sleep Time:	

BLOOD PRESSURE & WEIGHT

Time	SYS/DIA	Pulse

WEIGHT:

NOTES/SCHEDULE

7 am
8 am
9 am
10 am
11 am
12 pm
1 pm
2 pm
3 pm
4 pm
5 pm
6 pm
7 pm
8 pm

DATE: .... | SU | MO | TU | WE | TH | FR | SA

Month/Week: ....

FOOD, NUTRITION & MEDS

	Carbs	Sugars	Fiber	Protein	Fat	Calories
BREAKFAST Time: .... Meds/Insulin						
Breakfast Total						
SNACK 1 Time: .... Meds/Insulin						
Snack 1 Total						
LUNCH Time: .... Meds/Insulin						
Lunch Total						
SNACK 2 Time: .... Meds/Insulin						
Snack 2 Total						
DINNER Time: .... Meds/Insulin						
Dinner Total						
Total Nutrition for the Day						

Water Consumption ⊔ ⊔ ⊔ ⊔ ⊔ ⊔ ⊔ ⊔ ⊔ ⊔ ....

EXERCISE & ACTIVITY LOG

	Time/Duration	Intensity/Calories

BLOOD SUGAR LOG

	Blood Sugar Level	
	Before	After
WAKING-UP Time:	Sleep Hrs: .... Fast. Hrs :	
BREAKFAST		
SNACK 1		
LUNCH		
SNACK 2		
DINNER		
BEDTIME	Go to Sleep Time:	

BLOOD PRESSURE & WEIGHT

Time	SYS/DIA	Pulse

WEIGHT:

NOTES/SCHEDULE

7 am ....
8 am ....
9 am ....
10 am ....
11 am ....
12 pm ....
1 pm ....
2 pm ....
3 pm ....
4 pm ....
5 pm ....
6 pm ....
7 pm ....
8 pm ....

DATE:

| SU | MO | TU | WE | TH | FR | SA |

Month/ Week:

FOOD, NUTRITION & MEDS

	Carbs	Sugars	Fiber	Protein	Fat	Calories
BREAKFAST Time: .... Meds/Insulin						
Breakfast Total						
SNACK 1 Time: .... Meds/Insulin						
Snack 1 Total						
LUNCH Time: .... Meds/Insulin						
Lunch Total						
SNACK 2 Time: .... Meds/Insulin						
Snack 2 Total						
DINNER Time: .... Meds/Insulin						
Dinner Total						
Total Nutrition for the Day						

Water Consumption 🥛🥛🥛🥛 🥛🥛🥛🥛🥛🥛

EXERCISE & ACTIVITY LOG

	Time/Duration	Intensity/Calories

BLOOD SUGAR LOG

	Blood Sugar Level	
	Before	After
WAKING-UP Time:	Sleep Hrs: Fast. Hrs :	
BREAKFAST		
SNACK 1		
LUNCH		
SNACK 2		
DINNER		
BEDTIME	Go to Sleep Time:	

BLOOD PRESSURE & WEIGHT

Time	SYS/DIA	Pulse
WEIGHT:		

NOTES/SCHEDULE

7 am

8 am

9 am

10 am

11 am

12 pm

1 pm

2 pm

3 pm

4 pm

5 pm

6 pm

7 pm

8 pm

| DATE: | | SU | MO | TU | WE | TH | FR | SA | | **Month/ Week:** |

FOOD, NUTRITION & MEDS

	Carbs	Sugars	Fiber	Protein	Fat	Calories
BREAKFAST Time:	Meds/ Insulin					
Breakfast Total						
SNACK 1 Time:	Meds/ Insulin					
Snack 1 Total						
LUNCH Time:	Meds/ Insulin					
Lunch Total						
SNACK 2 Time:	Meds/ Insulin					
Snack 2 Total						
DINNER Time:	Meds/ Insulin					
Dinner Total						
Total Nutrition for the Day						

Water Consumption

EXERCISE & ACTIVITY LOG

	Time/Duration	Intensity/Calories

BLOOD SUGAR LOG

	Blood Sugar Level	
	Before	After
WAKING-UP Time:	Sleep Hrs: Fast. Hrs :	
BREAKFAST		
SNACK 1		
LUNCH		
SNACK 2		
DINNER		
BEDTIME	Go to Sleep Time:	

BLOOD PRESSURE & WEIGHT

Time	SYS/DIA	Pulse
WEIGHT:		

NOTES/SCHEDULE

7 am
8 am
9 am
10 am
11 am
12 pm
1 pm
2 pm
3 pm
4 pm
5 pm
6 pm
7 pm
8 pm

DATE: .... | SU | MO | TU | WE | TH | FR | SA

Month/Week: ....

FOOD, NUTRITION & MEDS

	Carbs	Sugars	Fiber	Protein	Fat	Calories
BREAKFAST Time: .... Meds/Insulin						
Breakfast Total						
SNACK 1 Time: .... Meds/Insulin						
Snack 1 Total						
LUNCH Time: .... Meds/Insulin						
Lunch Total						
SNACK 2 Time: .... Meds/Insulin						
Snack 2 Total						
DINNER Time: .... Meds/Insulin						
Dinner Total						
Total Nutrition for the Day						

Water Consumption ⬜⬜⬜⬜⬜⬜⬜⬜⬜

EXERCISE & ACTIVITY LOG

	Time/Duration	Intensity/Calories

BLOOD SUGAR LOG

	Blood Sugar Level	
	Before	After
WAKING-UP Time:	Sleep Hrs: .... Fast. Hrs :	
BREAKFAST		
SNACK 1		
LUNCH		
SNACK 2		
DINNER		
BEDTIME	Go to Sleep Time:	

BLOOD PRESSURE & WEIGHT

Time	SYS/DIA	Pulse

WEIGHT:

NOTES/SCHEDULE

7 am
8 am
9 am
10 am
11 am
12 pm
1 pm
2 pm
3 pm
4 pm
5 pm
6 pm
7 pm
8 pm

DATE:	SU	MO	TU	WE	TH	FR	SA	Month/ Week:

FOOD, NUTRITION & MEDS

	Carbs	Sugars	Fiber	Protein	Fat	Calories
BREAKFAST Time:	Meds/ Insulin					
Breakfast Total						
SNACK 1 Time:	Meds/ Insulin					
Snack 1 Total						
LUNCH Time:	Meds/ Insulin					
Lunch Total						
SNACK 2 Time:	Meds/ Insulin					
Snack 2 Total						
DINNER Time:	Meds/ Insulin					
Dinner Total						
Total Nutrition for the Day						

Water Consumption ▢ ▢ ▢ ▢ ▢ ▢ ▢ ▢ ▢ ▢ ....

EXERCISE & ACTIVITY LOG

	Time/Duration	Intensity/Calories

BLOOD SUGAR LOG

	Blood Sugar Level	
	Before	After
WAKING-UP Time:	Sleep Hrs: Fast. Hrs :	
BREAKFAST		
SNACK 1		
LUNCH		
SNACK 2		
DINNER		
BEDTIME	Go to Sleep Time:	

BLOOD PRESSURE & WEIGHT

Time	SYS/DIA	Pulse

WEIGHT: ....

NOTES/SCHEDULE

7 am
8 am
9 am
10 am
11 am
12 pm
1 pm
2 pm
3 pm
4 pm
5 pm
6 pm
7 pm
8 pm

DATE:	SU	MO	TU	WE	TH	FR	SA	Month/ Week:

FOOD, NUTRITION & MEDS

	Carbs	Sugars	Fiber	Protein	Fat	Calories
BREAKFAST Time:						
Meds/Insulin						
Breakfast Total						
SNACK 1 Time:						
Meds/Insulin						
Snack 1 Total						
LUNCH Time:						
Meds/Insulin						
Lunch Total						
SNACK 2 Time:						
Meds/Insulin						
Snack 2 Total						
DINNER Time:						
Meds/Insulin						
Dinner Total						
Total Nutrition for the Day						

Water Consumption ☐ ☐ ☐ ☐ ☐ ☐ ☐ ☐

EXERCISE & ACTIVITY LOG

	Time/Duration	Intensity/Calories

BLOOD SUGAR LOG

	Blood Sugar Level	
	Before	After
WAKING-UP Time:	Sleep Hrs: / Fast. Hrs :	
BREAKFAST		
SNACK 1		
LUNCH		
SNACK 2		
DINNER		
BEDTIME	Go to Sleep Time:	

BLOOD PRESSURE & WEIGHT

Time	SYS/DIA	Pulse

WEIGHT:

NOTES/SCHEDULE

7 am
8 am
9 am
10 am
11 am
12 pm
1 pm
2 pm
3 pm
4 pm
5 pm
6 pm
7 pm
8 pm

DATE:	SU	MO	TU	WE	TH	FR	SA	Month/ Week:	

FOOD, NUTRITION & MEDS

	Carbs	Sugars	Fiber	Protein	Fat	Calories
BREAKFAST Time: .... Meds/ Insulin						
Breakfast Total						
SNACK 1 Time: .... Meds/ Insulin						
Snack 1 Total						
LUNCH Time: .... Meds/ Insulin						
Lunch Total						
SNACK 2 Time: .... Meds/ Insulin						
Snack 2 Total						
DINNER Time: .... Meds/ Insulin						
Dinner Total						
Total Nutrition for the Day						

Water Consumption ⎕⎕⎕⎕⎕⎕⎕⎕⎕⎕ ....

EXERCISE & ACTIVITY LOG

	Time/Duration	Intensity/Calories

BLOOD SUGAR LOG

	Blood Sugar Level	
	Before	After
WAKING-UP Time:	Sleep Hrs: Fast. Hrs :	
BREAKFAST		
SNACK 1		
LUNCH		
SNACK 2		
DINNER		
BEDTIME	Go to Sleep Time:	

BLOOD PRESSURE & WEIGHT

Time	SYS/DIA	Pulse
WEIGHT:		

NOTES/SCHEDULE

7 am
8 am
9 am
10 am
11 am
12 pm
1 pm
2 pm
3 pm
4 pm
5 pm
6 pm
7 pm
8 pm

DATE:	SU	MO	TU	WE	TH	FR	SA		Month/ Week:

FOOD, NUTRITION & MEDS

	Carbs	Sugars	Fiber	Protein	Fat	Calories
BREAKFAST Time: _____ Meds/Insulin _____						
Breakfast Total						
SNACK 1 Time: _____ Meds/Insulin _____						
Snack 1 Total						
LUNCH Time: _____ Meds/Insulin _____						
Lunch Total						
SNACK 2 Time: _____ Meds/Insulin _____						
Snack 2 Total						
DINNER Time: _____ Meds/Insulin _____						
Dinner Total						
Total Nutrition for the Day						

Water Consumption 🥛🥛🥛🥛🥛🥛🥛🥛🥛

EXERCISE & ACTIVITY LOG

	Time/Duration	Intensity/Calories

BLOOD SUGAR LOG

	Blood Sugar Level	
	Before	After
WAKING-UP Time: _____	Sleep Hrs: _____ Fast. Hrs : _____	
BREAKFAST		
SNACK 1		
LUNCH		
SNACK 2		
DINNER		
BEDTIME	Go to Sleep Time: _____	

BLOOD PRESSURE & WEIGHT

Time	SYS/DIA	Pulse

WEIGHT: _____

NOTES/SCHEDULE

7 am
8 am
9 am
10 am
11 am
12 pm
1 pm
2 pm
3 pm
4 pm
5 pm
6 pm
7 pm
8 pm

DATE:		SU	MO	TU	WE	TH	FR	SA		Month/ Week:

FOOD, NUTRITION & MEDS

	Carbs	Sugars	Fiber	Protein	Fat	Calories
BREAKFAST Time: _____ Meds/Insulin						
Breakfast Total						
SNACK 1 Time: _____ Meds/Insulin						
Snack 1 Total						
LUNCH Time: _____ Meds/Insulin						
Lunch Total						
SNACK 2 Time: _____ Meds/Insulin						
Snack 2 Total						
DINNER Time: _____ Meds/Insulin						
Dinner Total						
Total Nutrition for the Day						

Water Consumption 🥛🥛🥛🥛🥛🥛🥛🥛🥛🥛 ....

EXERCISE & ACTIVITY LOG

	Time/Duration	Intensity/Calories

BLOOD SUGAR LOG

	Blood Sugar Level	
	Before	After
WAKING-UP Time:	Sleep Hrs: _____ Fast. Hrs :	
BREAKFAST		
SNACK 1		
LUNCH		
SNACK 2		
DINNER		
BEDTIME	Go to Sleep Time:	

BLOOD PRESSURE & WEIGHT

Time	SYS/DIA	Pulse

WEIGHT: ....

NOTES/SCHEDULE

7 am
8 am
9 am
10 am
11 am
12 pm
1 pm
2 pm
3 pm
4 pm
5 pm
6 pm
7 pm
8 pm

DATE: | SU | MO | TU | WE | TH | FR | SA

Month/Week: ....

FOOD, NUTRITION & MEDS

	Carbs	Sugars	Fiber	Protein	Fat	Calories

BREAKFAST Time: ....

Meds/Insulin ....

Breakfast Total

SNACK 1 Time: ....

Meds/Insulin ....

Snack 1 Total

LUNCH Time: ....

Meds/Insulin ....

Lunch Total

SNACK 2 Time: ....

Meds/Insulin ....

Snack 2 Total

DINNER Time: ....

Meds/Insulin ....

Dinner Total

Total Nutrition for the Day

Water Consumption ⬜⬜⬜⬜⬜⬜⬜⬜⬜ ....

EXERCISE & ACTIVITY LOG

	Time/Duration	Intensity/Calories

BLOOD SUGAR LOG

	Blood Sugar Level	
	Before	After
WAKING-UP Time:	Sleep Hrs: Fast. Hrs :	
BREAKFAST		
SNACK 1		
LUNCH		
SNACK 2		
DINNER		
BEDTIME	Go to Sleep Time:	

BLOOD PRESSURE & WEIGHT

Time	SYS/DIA	Pulse

WEIGHT:

NOTES/SCHEDULE

7 am

8 am

9 am

10 am

11 am

12 pm

1 pm

2 pm

3 pm

4 pm

5 pm

6 pm

7 pm

8 pm

DATE:		SU	MO	TU	WE	TH	FR	SA		**Month/Week:**

FOOD, NUTRITION & MEDS

	Carbs	Sugars	Fiber	Protein	Fat	Calories
BREAKFAST Time: .... Meds/Insulin						
Breakfast Total						
SNACK 1 Time: .... Meds/Insulin						
Snack 1 Total						
LUNCH Time: .... Meds/Insulin						
Lunch Total						
SNACK 2 Time: .... Meds/Insulin						
Snack 2 Total						
DINNER Time: .... Meds/Insulin						
Dinner Total						
Total Nutrition for the Day						

Water Consumption ☐ ☐ ☐ ☐ ☐ ☐ ☐ ☐ ☐ ☐ ....

EXERCISE & ACTIVITY LOG

	Time/Duration	Intensity/Calories

BLOOD SUGAR LOG

	Blood Sugar Level	
	Before	After
WAKING-UP Time:	Sleep Hrs: Fast. Hrs :	
BREAKFAST		
SNACK 1		
LUNCH		
SNACK 2		
DINNER		
BEDTIME	Go to Sleep Time:	

BLOOD PRESSURE & WEIGHT

Time	SYS/DIA	Pulse

WEIGHT: ....

NOTES/SCHEDULE

7 am
8 am
9 am
10 am
11 am
12 pm
1 pm
2 pm
3 pm
4 pm
5 pm
6 pm
7 pm
8 pm

DATE: .... | SU | MO | TU | WE | TH | FR | SA | **Month/ Week:** ....

FOOD, NUTRITION & MEDS

	Carbs	Sugars	Fiber	Protein	Fat	Calories
BREAKFAST Time: .... Meds/ Insulin						
Breakfast Total						
SNACK 1 Time: .... Meds/ Insulin						
Snack 1 Total						
LUNCH Time: .... Meds/ Insulin						
Lunch Total						
SNACK 2 Time: .... Meds/ Insulin						
Snack 2 Total						
DINNER Time: .... Meds/ Insulin						
Dinner Total						
Total Nutrition for the Day						

Water Consumption ▢▢▢▢▢▢▢▢▢ ....

EXERCISE & ACTIVITY LOG

	Time/Duration	Intensity/Calories

BLOOD SUGAR LOG

	Blood Sugar Level	
	Before	After
WAKING-UP Time:	Sleep Hrs: Fast. Hrs :	
BREAKFAST		
SNACK 1		
LUNCH		
SNACK 2		
DINNER		
BEDTIME	Go to Sleep Time:	

BLOOD PRESSURE & WEIGHT

Time	SYS/DIA	Pulse

WEIGHT:

NOTES/SCHEDULE

7 am
8 am
9 am
10 am
11 am
12 pm
1 pm
2 pm
3 pm
4 pm
5 pm
6 pm
7 pm
8 pm

DATE:	SU	MO	TU	WE	TH	FR	SA	Month/ Week:

FOOD, NUTRITION & MEDS

	Carbs	Sugars	Fiber	Protein	Fat	Calories
BREAKFAST Time: .... Meds/Insulin						
Breakfast Total						
SNACK 1 Time: .... Meds/Insulin						
Snack 1 Total						
LUNCH Time: .... Meds/Insulin						
Lunch Total						
SNACK 2 Time: .... Meds/Insulin						
Snack 2 Total						
DINNER Time: .... Meds/Insulin						
Dinner Total						
Total Nutrition for the Day						

Water Consumption 🥛🥛🥛🥛🥛🥛🥛🥛🥛🥛

EXERCISE & ACTIVITY LOG

	Time/Duration	Intensity/Calories

BLOOD SUGAR LOG

	Blood Sugar Level	
	Before	After
WAKING-UP Time:	Sleep Hrs: / Fast. Hrs :	
BREAKFAST		
SNACK 1		
LUNCH		
SNACK 2		
DINNER		
BEDTIME	Go to Sleep Time:	

BLOOD PRESSURE & WEIGHT

Time	SYS/DIA	Pulse

WEIGHT:

NOTES/SCHEDULE

7 am
8 am
9 am
10 am
11 am
12 pm
1 pm
2 pm
3 pm
4 pm
5 pm
6 pm
7 pm
8 pm

DATE: | SU | MO | TU | WE | TH | FR | SA

Month/ Week:

FOOD, NUTRITION & MEDS

	Carbs	Sugars	Fiber	Protein	Fat	Calories
BREAKFAST Time:	Meds/ Insulin					
Breakfast Total						
SNACK 1 Time:	Meds/ Insulin					
Snack 1 Total						
LUNCH Time:	Meds/ Insulin					
Lunch Total						
SNACK 2 Time:	Meds/ Insulin					
Snack 2 Total						
DINNER Time:	Meds/ Insulin					
Dinner Total						
Total Nutrition for the Day						

Water Consumption

EXERCISE & ACTIVITY LOG

	Time/Duration	Intensity/Calories

BLOOD SUGAR LOG

	Blood Sugar Level	
	Before	After
WAKING-UP Time:	Sleep Hrs: Fast. Hrs :	
BREAKFAST		
SNACK 1		
LUNCH		
SNACK 2		
DINNER		
BEDTIME	Go to Sleep Time:	

BLOOD PRESSURE & WEIGHT

Time	SYS/DIA	Pulse

WEIGHT:

NOTES/SCHEDULE

7 am
8 am
9 am
10 am
11 am
12 pm
1 pm
2 pm
3 pm
4 pm
5 pm
6 pm
7 pm
8 pm

DATE:	SU	MO	TU	WE	TH	FR	SA	Month/ Week:

FOOD, NUTRITION & MEDS

	Carbs	Sugars	Fiber	Protein	Fat	Calories
BREAKFAST Time: Meds/Insulin						
Breakfast Total						
SNACK 1 Time: Meds/Insulin						
Snack 1 Total						
LUNCH Time: Meds/Insulin						
Lunch Total						
SNACK 2 Time: Meds/Insulin						
Snack 2 Total						
DINNER Time: Meds/Insulin						
Dinner Total						
Total Nutrition for the Day						

Water Consumption ⊔⊔⊔⊔⊔⊔⊔⊔⊔⊔ ....

EXERCISE & ACTIVITY LOG

	Time/Duration	Intensity/Calories

BLOOD SUGAR LOG

	Blood Sugar Level	
	Before	After
WAKING-UP Time:	Sleep Hrs: Fast. Hrs :	
BREAKFAST		
SNACK 1		
LUNCH		
SNACK 2		
DINNER		
BEDTIME	Go to Sleep Time:	

BLOOD PRESSURE & WEIGHT

Time	SYS/DIA	Pulse

WEIGHT:

NOTES/SCHEDULE

7 am
8 am
9 am
10 am
11 am
12 pm
1 pm
2 pm
3 pm
4 pm
5 pm
6 pm
7 pm
8 pm

DATE:		SU	MO	TU	WE	TH	FR	SA	Month/ Week:

FOOD, NUTRITION & MEDS

	Carbs	Sugars	Fiber	Protein	Fat	Calories
BREAKFAST Time:	Meds/ Insulin					
Breakfast Total						
SNACK 1 Time:	Meds/ Insulin					
Snack 1 Total						
LUNCH Time:	Meds/ Insulin					
Lunch Total						
SNACK 2 Time:	Meds/ Insulin					
Snack 2 Total						
DINNER Time:	Meds/ Insulin					
Dinner Total						
Total Nutrition for the Day						

Water Consumption ☐ ☐ ☐ ☐ ☐ ☐ ☐ ☐ ☐

EXERCISE & ACTIVITY LOG

	Time/Duration	Intensity/Calories

BLOOD SUGAR LOG

	Blood Sugar Level	
	Before	After
WAKING-UP Time:	Sleep Hrs: Fast. Hrs :	
BREAKFAST		
SNACK 1		
LUNCH		
SNACK 2		
DINNER		
BEDTIME	Go to Sleep Time:	

BLOOD PRESSURE & WEIGHT

Time	SYS/DIA	Pulse

WEIGHT:

NOTES/SCHEDULE

7 am
8 am
9 am
10 am
11 am
12 pm
1 pm
2 pm
3 pm
4 pm
5 pm
6 pm
7 pm
8 pm

DATE: | SU | MO | TU | WE | TH | FR | SA

Month/ Week: ....

FOOD, NUTRITION & MEDS

		Carbs	Sugars	Fiber	Protein	Fat	Calories
BREAKFAST Time:	Meds/ Insulin						
Breakfast Total							
SNACK 1 Time:	Meds/ Insulin						
Snack 1 Total							
LUNCH Time:	Meds/ Insulin						
Lunch Total							
SNACK 2 Time:	Meds/ Insulin						
Snack 2 Total							
DINNER Time:	Meds/ Insulin						
Dinner Total							
Total Nutrition for the Day							

Water Consumption ▭ ▭ ▭ ▭ ▭ ▭ ▭ ▭ ▭ ▭ ....

EXERCISE & ACTIVITY LOG

	Time/Duration	Intensity/Calories

BLOOD SUGAR LOG

	Blood Sugar Level	
	Before	After
WAKING-UP Time:	Sleep Hrs: Fast. Hrs :	
BREAKFAST		
SNACK 1		
LUNCH		
SNACK 2		
DINNER		
BEDTIME	Go to Sleep Time:	

BLOOD PRESSURE & WEIGHT

Time	SYS/DIA	Pulse

WEIGHT:

NOTES/SCHEDULE

7 am
8 am
9 am
10 am
11 am
12 pm
1 pm
2 pm
3 pm
4 pm
5 pm
6 pm
7 pm
8 pm

DATE: .... | SU | MO | TU | WE | TH | FR | SA

Month/ Week: ....

FOOD, NUTRITION & MEDS

	Carbs	Sugars	Fiber	Protein	Fat	Calories
BREAKFAST Time: .... Meds/Insulin						
Breakfast Total						
SNACK 1 Time: .... Meds/Insulin						
Snack 1 Total						
LUNCH Time: .... Meds/Insulin						
Lunch Total						
SNACK 2 Time: .... Meds/Insulin						
Snack 2 Total						
DINNER Time: .... Meds/Insulin						
Dinner Total						
Total Nutrition for the Day						

Water Consumption ⬜⬜⬜⬜⬜⬜⬜⬜ ....

EXERCISE & ACTIVITY LOG

	Time/Duration	Intensity/Calories

BLOOD SUGAR LOG

	Blood Sugar Level	
	Before	After
WAKING-UP Time:	Sleep Hrs: Fast. Hrs :	
BREAKFAST		
SNACK 1		
LUNCH		
SNACK 2		
DINNER		
BEDTIME	Go to Sleep Time:	

BLOOD PRESSURE & WEIGHT

Time	SYS/DIA	Pulse

WEIGHT:

NOTES/SCHEDULE

7 am
8 am
9 am
10 am
11 am
12 pm
1 pm
2 pm
3 pm
4 pm
5 pm
6 pm
7 pm
8 pm

DATE:	SU	MO	TU	WE	TH	FR	SA	Month/ Week:

FOOD, NUTRITION & MEDS

	Carbs	Sugars	Fiber	Protein	Fat	Calories
BREAKFAST Time: .... Meds/Insulin						
Breakfast Total						
SNACK 1 Time: .... Meds/Insulin						
Snack 1 Total						
LUNCH Time: .... Meds/Insulin						
Lunch Total						
SNACK 2 Time: .... Meds/Insulin						
Snack 2 Total						
DINNER Time: .... Meds/Insulin						
Dinner Total						
Total Nutrition for the Day						

Water Consumption ⬜⬜⬜⬜⬜⬜⬜⬜⬜⬜ ....

EXERCISE & ACTIVITY LOG

	Time/Duration	Intensity/Calories

BLOOD SUGAR LOG

	Blood Sugar Level	
	Before	After
WAKING-UP Time:	Sleep Hrs: Fast. Hrs :	
BREAKFAST		
SNACK 1		
LUNCH		
SNACK 2		
DINNER		
BEDTIME	Go to Sleep Time:	

BLOOD PRESSURE & WEIGHT

Time	SYS/DIA	Pulse
WEIGHT:		

NOTES/SCHEDULE

7 am
8 am
9 am
10 am
11 am
12 pm
1 pm
2 pm
3 pm
4 pm
5 pm
6 pm
7 pm
8 pm

DATE:	SU	MO	TU	WE	TH	FR	SA		Month/ Week:

FOOD, NUTRITION & MEDS

	Carbs	Sugars	Fiber	Protein	Fat	Calories
BREAKFAST Time:	Meds/ Insulin					
Breakfast Total						
SNACK 1 Time:	Meds/ Insulin					
Snack 1 Total						
LUNCH Time:	Meds/ Insulin					
Lunch Total						
SNACK 2 Time:	Meds/ Insulin					
Snack 2 Total						
DINNER Time:	Meds/ Insulin					
Dinner Total						
Total Nutrition for the Day						

Water Consumption ⊔ ⊔ ⊔ ⊔ ⊔ ⊔ ⊔ ⊔ ⊔

EXERCISE & ACTIVITY LOG

	Time/Duration	Intensity/Calories

BLOOD SUGAR LOG

	Blood Sugar Level	
	Before	After
WAKING-UP Time:	Sleep Hrs: Fast. Hrs :	
BREAKFAST		
SNACK 1		
LUNCH		
SNACK 2		
DINNER		
BEDTIME	Go to Sleep Time:	

BLOOD PRESSURE & WEIGHT

Time	SYS/DIA	Pulse

WEIGHT:

NOTES/SCHEDULE

7 am
8 am
9 am
10 am
11 am
12 pm
1 pm
2 pm
3 pm
4 pm
5 pm
6 pm
7 pm
8 pm

DATE:	SU	MO	TU	WE	TH	FR	SA	Month/ Week:

FOOD, NUTRITION & MEDS

	Carbs	Sugars	Fiber	Protein	Fat	Calories
BREAKFAST Time: .... Meds/Insulin						
Breakfast Total						
SNACK 1 Time: .... Meds/Insulin						
Snack 1 Total						
LUNCH Time: .... Meds/Insulin						
Lunch Total						
SNACK 2 Time: .... Meds/Insulin						
Snack 2 Total						
DINNER Time: .... Meds/Insulin						
Dinner Total						
Total Nutrition for the Day						

Water Consumption ⬛⬛⬛⬛⬛⬛⬛⬛⬛⬛ ....

EXERCISE & ACTIVITY LOG

	Time/Duration	Intensity/Calories

BLOOD SUGAR LOG

	Blood Sugar Level	
	Before	After
WAKING-UP Time:	Sleep Hrs: .... Fast. Hrs :	
BREAKFAST		
SNACK 1		
LUNCH		
SNACK 2		
DINNER		
BEDTIME	Go to Sleep Time:	

BLOOD PRESSURE & WEIGHT

Time	SYS/DIA	Pulse

WEIGHT:

NOTES/SCHEDULE

7 am
8 am
9 am
10 am
11 am
12 pm
1 pm
2 pm
3 pm
4 pm
5 pm
6 pm
7 pm
8 pm

| DATE: | SU | MO | TU | WE | TH | FR | SA | Month/ Week: |

FOOD, NUTRITION & MEDS

	Carbs	Sugars	Fiber	Protein	Fat	Calories
BREAKFAST Time: — Meds/ Insulin						
Breakfast Total						
SNACK 1 Time: — Meds/ Insulin						
Snack 1 Total						
LUNCH Time: — Meds/ Insulin						
Lunch Total						
SNACK 2 Time: — Meds/ Insulin						
Snack 2 Total						
DINNER Time: — Meds/ Insulin						
Dinner Total						
Total Nutrition for the Day						

Water Consumption ▢ ▢ ▢ ▢ ▢ ▢ ▢ ▢ ▢

EXERCISE & ACTIVITY LOG

	Time/Duration	Intensity/Calories

BLOOD SUGAR LOG

	Blood Sugar Level	
	Before	After
WAKING-UP Time:	Sleep Hrs: Fast. Hrs :	
BREAKFAST		
SNACK 1		
LUNCH		
SNACK 2		
DINNER		
BEDTIME	Go to Sleep Time:	

BLOOD PRESSURE & WEIGHT

Time	SYS/DIA	Pulse

WEIGHT:

NOTES/SCHEDULE

7 am
8 am
9 am
10 am
11 am
12 pm
1 pm
2 pm
3 pm
4 pm
5 pm
6 pm
7 pm
8 pm

DATE:	SU	MO	TU	WE	TH	FR	SA	Month/ Week: ....

FOOD, NUTRITION & MEDS

	Carbs	Sugars	Fiber	Protein	Fat	Calories
BREAKFAST Time: .... Meds/Insulin						
Breakfast Total						
SNACK 1 Time: .... Meds/Insulin						
Snack 1 Total						
LUNCH Time: .... Meds/Insulin						
Lunch Total						
SNACK 2 Time: .... Meds/Insulin						
Snack 2 Total						
DINNER Time: .... Meds/Insulin						
Dinner Total						
Total Nutrition for the Day						

Water Consumption ▢ ▢ ▢ ▢ ▢ ▢ ▢ ▢ ▢ ....

EXERCISE & ACTIVITY LOG

	Time/Duration	Intensity/Calories

BLOOD SUGAR LOG

	Blood Sugar Level	
	Before	After
WAKING-UP Time:	Sleep Hrs: .... Fast. Hrs :	
BREAKFAST		
SNACK 1		
LUNCH		
SNACK 2		
DINNER		
BEDTIME	Go to Sleep Time:	

BLOOD PRESSURE & WEIGHT

Time	SYS/DIA	Pulse

WEIGHT: ....

NOTES/SCHEDULE

7 am
8 am
9 am
10 am
11 am
12 pm
1 pm
2 pm
3 pm
4 pm
5 pm
6 pm
7 pm
8 pm

DATE: .... | SU | MO | TU | WE | TH | FR | SA | **Month/ Week:** ....

FOOD, NUTRITION & MEDS

	Carbs	Sugars	Fiber	Protein	Fat	Calories
BREAKFAST Time: .... Meds/Insulin						
Breakfast Total						
SNACK 1 Time: .... Meds/Insulin						
Snack 1 Total						
LUNCH Time: .... Meds/Insulin						
Lunch Total						
SNACK 2 Time: .... Meds/Insulin						
Snack 2 Total						
DINNER Time: .... Meds/Insulin						
Dinner Total						
Total Nutrition for the Day						

Water Consumption ▢ ▢ ▢ ▢ ▢ ▢ ▢ ▢ ▢

EXERCISE & ACTIVITY LOG

	Time/Duration	Intensity/Calories

BLOOD SUGAR LOG

	Blood Sugar Level	
	Before	After
WAKING-UP Time:	Sleep Hrs: Fast. Hrs :	
BREAKFAST		
SNACK 1		
LUNCH		
SNACK 2		
DINNER		
BEDTIME	Go to Sleep Time:	

BLOOD PRESSURE & WEIGHT

Time	SYS/DIA	Pulse

WEIGHT:

NOTES/SCHEDULE

7 am
8 am
9 am
10 am
11 am
12 pm
1 pm
2 pm
3 pm
4 pm
5 pm
6 pm
7 pm
8 pm

DATE:	SU	MO	TU	WE	TH	FR	SA	Month/ Week:

FOOD, NUTRITION & MEDS

	Carbs	Sugars	Fiber	Protein	Fat	Calories
BREAKFAST Time:	Meds/ Insulin					
Breakfast Total						
SNACK 1 Time:	Meds/ Insulin					
Snack 1 Total						
LUNCH Time:	Meds/ Insulin					
Lunch Total						
SNACK 2 Time:	Meds/ Insulin					
Snack 2 Total						
DINNER Time:	Meds/ Insulin					
Dinner Total						
Total Nutrition for the Day						

Water Consumption 🥛 🥛 🥛 🥛 🥛 🥛 🥛 🥛 🥛 🥛

EXERCISE & ACTIVITY LOG

	Time/Duration	Intensity/Calories

BLOOD SUGAR LOG

	Blood Sugar Level	
	Before	After
WAKING-UP Time:	Sleep Hrs: Fast. Hrs :	
BREAKFAST		
SNACK 1		
LUNCH		
SNACK 2		
DINNER		
BEDTIME	Go to Sleep Time:	

BLOOD PRESSURE & WEIGHT

Time	SYS/DIA	Pulse
WEIGHT:		

NOTES/SCHEDULE

7 am
8 am
9 am
10 am
11 am
12 pm
1 pm
2 pm
3 pm
4 pm
5 pm
6 pm
7 pm
8 pm

DATE:		SU	MO	TU	WE	TH	FR	SA	Month/ Week:

FOOD, NUTRITION & MEDS

	Carbs	Sugars	Fiber	Protein	Fat	Calories
BREAKFAST Time: .... Meds/ Insulin						
Breakfast Total						
SNACK 1 Time: .... Meds/ Insulin						
Snack 1 Total						
LUNCH Time: .... Meds/ Insulin						
Lunch Total						
SNACK 2 Time: .... Meds/ Insulin						
Snack 2 Total						
DINNER Time: .... Meds/ Insulin						
Dinner Total						
Total Nutrition for the Day						

Water Consumption ▢ ▢ ▢ ▢ ▢ ▢ ▢ ▢ ▢ ....

EXERCISE & ACTIVITY LOG

	Time/Duration	Intensity/Calories

BLOOD SUGAR LOG

	Blood Sugar Level	
	Before	After
WAKING-UP Time:	Sleep Hrs: Fast. Hrs :	
BREAKFAST		
SNACK 1		
LUNCH		
SNACK 2		
DINNER		
BEDTIME	Go to Sleep Time:	

BLOOD PRESSURE & WEIGHT

Time	SYS/DIA	Pulse
WEIGHT:		

NOTES/SCHEDULE

7 am
8 am
9 am
10 am
11 am
12 pm
1 pm
2 pm
3 pm
4 pm
5 pm
6 pm
7 pm
8 pm

DATE:	SU	MO	TU	WE	TH	FR	SA	Month/ Week: ....

FOOD, NUTRITION & MEDS

	Carbs	Sugars	Fiber	Protein	Fat	Calories
BREAKFAST Time: .... Meds/Insulin						
Breakfast Total						
SNACK 1 Time: .... Meds/Insulin						
Snack 1 Total						
LUNCH Time: .... Meds/Insulin						
Lunch Total						
SNACK 2 Time: .... Meds/Insulin						
Snack 2 Total						
DINNER Time: .... Meds/Insulin						
Dinner Total						
Total Nutrition for the Day						

Water Consumption ⬜⬜⬜⬜⬜⬜⬜⬜⬜⬜ ....

EXERCISE & ACTIVITY LOG

	Time/Duration	Intensity/Calories

BLOOD SUGAR LOG

	Blood Sugar Level	
	Before	After
WAKING-UP Time:	Sleep Hrs: .... Fast. Hrs :	
BREAKFAST		
SNACK 1		
LUNCH		
SNACK 2		
DINNER		
BEDTIME	Go to Sleep Time:	

BLOOD PRESSURE & WEIGHT

Time	SYS/DIA	Pulse

WEIGHT:

NOTES/SCHEDULE

7 am
8 am
9 am
10 am
11 am
12 pm
1 pm
2 pm
3 pm
4 pm
5 pm
6 pm
7 pm
8 pm

DATE: .... | SU | MO | TU | WE | TH | FR | SA | **Month/ Week:** ....

FOOD, NUTRITION & MEDS

	Carbs	Sugars	Fiber	Protein	Fat	Calories
BREAKFAST Time: .... Meds/Insulin						
Breakfast Total						
SNACK 1 Time: .... Meds/Insulin						
Snack 1 Total						
LUNCH Time: .... Meds/Insulin						
Lunch Total						
SNACK 2 Time: .... Meds/Insulin						
Snack 2 Total						
DINNER Time: .... Meds/Insulin						
Dinner Total						
Total Nutrition for the Day						

Water Consumption 🥛🥛🥛🥛🥛🥛🥛🥛🥛

EXERCISE & ACTIVITY LOG

	Time/Duration	Intensity/Calories

BLOOD SUGAR LOG

	Blood Sugar Level	
	Before	After
WAKING-UP Time:	Sleep Hrs: Fast. Hrs :	
BREAKFAST		
SNACK 1		
LUNCH		
SNACK 2		
DINNER		
BEDTIME	Go to Sleep Time:	

BLOOD PRESSURE & WEIGHT

Time	SYS/DIA	Pulse

WEIGHT:

NOTES/SCHEDULE

7 am
8 am
9 am
10 am
11 am
12 pm
1 pm
2 pm
3 pm
4 pm
5 pm
6 pm
7 pm
8 pm

FOOD, NUTRITION & MEDS

	Carbs	Sugars	Fiber	Protein	Fat	Calories
BREAKFAST Time: .... Meds/Insulin						
Breakfast Total						
SNACK 1 Time: .... Meds/Insulin						
Snack 1 Total						
LUNCH Time: .... Meds/Insulin						
Lunch Total						
SNACK 2 Time: .... Meds/Insulin						
Snack 2 Total						
DINNER Time: .... Meds/Insulin						
Dinner Total						
Total Nutrition for the Day						

Water Consumption ☐ ☐ ☐ ☐ ☐ ☐ ☐ ☐ ☐ ☐ ....

EXERCISE & ACTIVITY LOG

	Time/Duration	Intensity/Calories

BLOOD SUGAR LOG

	Blood Sugar Level	
	Before	After
WAKING-UP Time:	Sleep Hrs: .... Fast. Hrs :	
BREAKFAST		
SNACK 1		
LUNCH		
SNACK 2		
DINNER		
BEDTIME	Go to Sleep Time:	

BLOOD PRESSURE & WEIGHT

Time	SYS/DIA	Pulse

WEIGHT:

NOTES/SCHEDULE

7 am
8 am
9 am
10 am
11 am
12 pm
1 pm
2 pm
3 pm
4 pm
5 pm
6 pm
7 pm
8 pm

DATE:	SU	MO	TU	WE	TH	FR	SA	Month/ Week:

FOOD, NUTRITION & MEDS

	Carbs	Sugars	Fiber	Protein	Fat	Calories
BREAKFAST Time: ____ Meds/ Insulin						
Breakfast Total						
SNACK 1 Time: ____ Meds/ Insulin						
Snack 1 Total						
LUNCH Time: ____ Meds/ Insulin						
Lunch Total						
SNACK 2 Time: ____ Meds/ Insulin						
Snack 2 Total						
DINNER Time: ____ Meds/ Insulin						
Dinner Total						
Total Nutrition for the Day						

Water Consumption ▭ ▭ ▭ ▭ ▭ ▭ ▭ ▭

EXERCISE & ACTIVITY LOG

	Time/Duration	Intensity/Calories

BLOOD SUGAR LOG

	Blood Sugar Level	
	Before	After
WAKING-UP Time:	Sleep Hrs: Fast. Hrs :	
BREAKFAST		
SNACK 1		
LUNCH		
SNACK 2		
DINNER		
BEDTIME	Go to Sleep Time:	

BLOOD PRESSURE & WEIGHT

Time	SYS/DIA	Pulse

WEIGHT: ____

NOTES/SCHEDULE

7 am
8 am
9 am
10 am
11 am
12 pm
1 pm
2 pm
3 pm
4 pm
5 pm
6 pm
7 pm
8 pm

DATE:	SU	MO	TU	WE	TH	FR	SA	Month/ Week:

FOOD, NUTRITION & MEDS

	Carbs	Sugars	Fiber	Protein	Fat	Calories
BREAKFAST Time:	Meds/ Insulin					
Breakfast Total						
SNACK 1 Time:	Meds/ Insulin					
Snack 1 Total						
LUNCH Time:	Meds/ Insulin					
Lunch Total						
SNACK 2 Time:	Meds/ Insulin					
Snack 2 Total						
DINNER Time:	Meds/ Insulin					
Dinner Total						
Total Nutrition for the Day						

Water Consumption ▢ ▢ ▢ ▢ ▢ ▢ ▢ ▢ ▢

EXERCISE & ACTIVITY LOG

	Time/Duration	Intensity/Calories

BLOOD SUGAR LOG

	Blood Sugar Level	
	Before	After
WAKING-UP Time:	Sleep Hrs: Fast. Hrs :	
BREAKFAST		
SNACK 1		
LUNCH		
SNACK 2		
DINNER		
BEDTIME	Go to Sleep Time:	

BLOOD PRESSURE & WEIGHT

Time	SYS/DIA	Pulse
WEIGHT:		

NOTES/SCHEDULE

7 am
8 am
9 am
10 am
11 am
12 pm
1 pm
2 pm
3 pm
4 pm
5 pm
6 pm
7 pm
8 pm

DATE:		SU	MO	TU	WE	TH	FR	SA	Month/ Week:

FOOD, NUTRITION & MEDS

	Carbs	Sugars	Fiber	Protein	Fat	Calories
BREAKFAST Time: .... Meds/Insulin						
Breakfast Total						
SNACK 1 Time: .... Meds/Insulin						
Snack 1 Total						
LUNCH Time: .... Meds/Insulin						
Lunch Total						
SNACK 2 Time: .... Meds/Insulin						
Snack 2 Total						
DINNER Time: .... Meds/Insulin						
Dinner Total						
Total Nutrition for the Day						

Water Consumption ▢ ▢ ▢ ▢ ▢ ▢ ▢ ▢ ▢ ....

EXERCISE & ACTIVITY LOG

	Time/Duration	Intensity/Calories
....	....	....
....	....	....
....	....	....
....	....	....

BLOOD SUGAR LOG

	Blood Sugar Level	
	Before	After
WAKING-UP Time:	Sleep Hrs: Fast. Hrs :	
BREAKFAST		
SNACK 1		
LUNCH		
SNACK 2		
DINNER		
BEDTIME	Go to Sleep Time:	

BLOOD PRESSURE & WEIGHT

Time	SYS/DIA	Pulse

WEIGHT:

NOTES/SCHEDULE

7 am
8 am
9 am
10 am
11 am
12 pm
1 pm
2 pm
3 pm
4 pm
5 pm
6 pm
7 pm
8 pm

FOOD, NUTRITION & MEDS

	Carbs	Sugars	Fiber	Protein	Fat	Calories
BREAKFAST Time: Meds/Insulin						
Breakfast Total						
SNACK 1 Time: Meds/Insulin						
Snack 1 Total						
LUNCH Time: Meds/Insulin						
Lunch Total						
SNACK 2 Time: Meds/Insulin						
Snack 2 Total						
DINNER Time: Meds/Insulin						
Dinner Total						
Total Nutrition for the Day						

Water Consumption ☐ ☐ ☐ ☐ ☐ ☐ ☐ ☐ ☐

EXERCISE & ACTIVITY LOG

	Time/Duration	Intensity/Calories

BLOOD SUGAR LOG

	Blood Sugar Level	
	Before	After
WAKING-UP Time:	Sleep Hrs: Fast. Hrs :	
BREAKFAST		
SNACK 1		
LUNCH		
SNACK 2		
DINNER		
BEDTIME	Go to Sleep Time:	

BLOOD PRESSURE & WEIGHT

Time	SYS/DIA	Pulse

WEIGHT:

NOTES/SCHEDULE

7 am
8 am
9 am
10 am
11 am
12 pm
1 pm
2 pm
3 pm
4 pm
5 pm
6 pm
7 pm
8 pm

FOOD, NUTRITION & MEDS

	Carbs	Sugars	Fiber	Protein	Fat	Calories

BREAKFAST   Time:

Meds/Insulin

Breakfast Total

SNACK 1   Time:

Meds/Insulin

Snack 1 Total

LUNCH   Time:

Meds/Insulin

Lunch Total

SNACK 2   Time:

Meds/Insulin

Snack 2 Total

DINNER   Time:

Meds/Insulin

Dinner Total

Total Nutrition for the Day

Water Consumption

EXERCISE & ACTIVITY LOG

	Time/Duration	Intensity/Calories

BLOOD SUGAR LOG

	Blood Sugar Level	
	Before	After
WAKING-UP Time:	Sleep Hrs: Fast. Hrs :	
BREAKFAST		
SNACK 1		
LUNCH		
SNACK 2		
DINNER		
BEDTIME	Go to Sleep Time:	

BLOOD PRESSURE & WEIGHT

Time	SYS/DIA	Pulse

WEIGHT:

NOTES/SCHEDULE

7 am
8 am
9 am
10 am
11 am
12 pm
1 pm
2 pm
3 pm
4 pm
5 pm
6 pm
7 pm
8 pm

DATE:		SU	MO	TU	WE	TH	FR	SA		Month/ Week:

FOOD, NUTRITION & MEDS

	Carbs	Sugars	Fiber	Protein	Fat	Calories
BREAKFAST Time:	Meds/ Insulin					
Breakfast Total						
SNACK 1 Time:	Meds/ Insulin					
Snack 1 Total						
LUNCH Time:	Meds/ Insulin					
Lunch Total						
SNACK 2 Time:	Meds/ Insulin					
Snack 2 Total						
DINNER Time:	Meds/ Insulin					
Dinner Total						
Total Nutrition for the Day						

Water Consumption

EXERCISE & ACTIVITY LOG

	Time/Duration	Intensity/Calories

BLOOD SUGAR LOG

	Blood Sugar Level	
	Before	After
WAKING-UP Time:	Sleep Hrs: Fast. Hrs :	
BREAKFAST		
SNACK 1		
LUNCH		
SNACK 2		
DINNER		
BEDTIME	Go to Sleep Time:	

BLOOD PRESSURE & WEIGHT

Time	SYS/DIA	Pulse
WEIGHT:		

NOTES/SCHEDULE

7 am
8 am
9 am
10 am
11 am
12 pm
1 pm
2 pm
3 pm
4 pm
5 pm
6 pm
7 pm
8 pm

DATE: ....   SU | MO | TU | WE | TH | FR | SA

Month/ Week: ....

FOOD, NUTRITION & MEDS

	Carbs	Sugars	Fiber	Protein	Fat	Calories
BREAKFAST Time: .... Meds/ Insulin						
Breakfast Total						
SNACK 1 Time: .... Meds/ Insulin						
Snack 1 Total						
LUNCH Time: .... Meds/ Insulin						
Lunch Total						
SNACK 2 Time: .... Meds/ Insulin						
Snack 2 Total						
DINNER Time: .... Meds/ Insulin						
Dinner Total						
Total Nutrition for the Day						

Water Consumption ▢ ▢ ▢ ▢ ▢ ▢ ▢ ▢ ▢

EXERCISE & ACTIVITY LOG

	Time/Duration	Intensity/Calories

BLOOD SUGAR LOG

	Blood Sugar Level	
	Before	After
WAKING-UP Time:	Sleep Hrs: .... Fast. Hrs :	
BREAKFAST		
SNACK 1		
LUNCH		
SNACK 2		
DINNER		
BEDTIME	Go to Sleep Time:	

BLOOD PRESSURE & WEIGHT

Time	SYS/DIA	Pulse

WEIGHT:

NOTES/SCHEDULE

7 am
8 am
9 am
10 am
11 am
12 pm
1 pm
2 pm
3 pm
4 pm
5 pm
6 pm
7 pm
8 pm

DATE: | SU | MO | TU | WE | TH | FR | SA

Month/Week: ....

FOOD, NUTRITION & MEDS

	Carbs	Sugars	Fiber	Protein	Fat	Calories

BREAKFAST Time: .... Meds/Insulin ....

Breakfast Total						

SNACK 1 Time: .... Meds/Insulin ....

Snack 1 Total						

LUNCH Time: .... Meds/Insulin ....

Lunch Total						

SNACK 2 Time: .... Meds/Insulin ....

Snack 2 Total						

DINNER Time: .... Meds/Insulin ....

Dinner Total						
Total Nutrition for the Day						

Water Consumption ⌷ ⌷ ⌷ ⌷ ⌷ ⌷ ⌷ ⌷

EXERCISE & ACTIVITY LOG

	Time/Duration	Intensity/Calories

BLOOD SUGAR LOG

	Blood Sugar Level	
	Before	After
WAKING-UP Time:	Sleep Hrs: .... Fast. Hrs :	
BREAKFAST		
SNACK 1		
LUNCH		
SNACK 2		
DINNER		
BEDTIME	Go to Sleep Time:	

BLOOD PRESSURE & WEIGHT

Time	SYS/DIA	Pulse
WEIGHT:		

NOTES/SCHEDULE

7 am
8 am
9 am
10 am
11 am
12 pm
1 pm
2 pm
3 pm
4 pm
5 pm
6 pm
7 pm
8 pm

DATE: .... | SU | MO | TU | WE | TH | FR | SA | **Month/ Week:** ....

FOOD, NUTRITION & MEDS

	Carbs	Sugars	Fiber	Protein	Fat	Calories
BREAKFAST Time: .... Meds/ Insulin						
Breakfast Total						
SNACK 1 Time: .... Meds/ Insulin						
Snack 1 Total						
LUNCH Time: .... Meds/ Insulin						
Lunch Total						
SNACK 2 Time: .... Meds/ Insulin						
Snack 2 Total						
DINNER Time: .... Meds/ Insulin						
Dinner Total						
Total Nutrition for the Day						

Water Consumption ▢ ▢ ▢ ▢ ▢ ▢ ▢ ▢ ▢

EXERCISE & ACTIVITY LOG

	Time/Duration	Intensity/Calories

BLOOD SUGAR LOG

	Blood Sugar Level	
	Before	After
WAKING-UP Time:	Sleep Hrs: Fast. Hrs :	
BREAKFAST		
SNACK 1		
LUNCH		
SNACK 2		
DINNER		
BEDTIME	Go to Sleep Time:	

BLOOD PRESSURE & WEIGHT

Time	SYS/DIA	Pulse

WEIGHT:

NOTES/SCHEDULE

7 am
8 am
9 am
10 am
11 am
12 pm
1 pm
2 pm
3 pm
4 pm
5 pm
6 pm
7 pm
8 pm

DATE:		SU	MO	TU	WE	TH	FR	SA		Month/ Week:

FOOD, NUTRITION & MEDS

	Carbs	Sugars	Fiber	Protein	Fat	Calories
BREAKFAST Time:						
Meds/ Insulin						
Breakfast Total						
SNACK 1 Time:						
Meds/ Insulin						
Snack 1 Total						
LUNCH Time:						
Meds/ Insulin						
Lunch Total						
SNACK 2 Time:						
Meds/ Insulin						
Snack 2 Total						
DINNER Time:						
Meds/ Insulin						
Dinner Total						
Total Nutrition for the Day						

Water Consumption ▢ ▢ ▢ ▢ ▢ ▢ ▢ ▢ ▢ ▢

EXERCISE & ACTIVITY LOG

	Time/Duration	Intensity/Calories

BLOOD SUGAR LOG

	Blood Sugar Level	
	Before	After
WAKING-UP Time:	Sleep Hrs: Fast. Hrs :	
BREAKFAST		
SNACK 1		
LUNCH		
SNACK 2		
DINNER		
BEDTIME	Go to Sleep Time:	

BLOOD PRESSURE & WEIGHT

Time	SYS/DIA	Pulse
WEIGHT:		

NOTES/SCHEDULE

7 am
8 am
9 am
10 am
11 am
12 pm
1 pm
2 pm
3 pm
4 pm
5 pm
6 pm
7 pm
8 pm

DATE: .... SU | MO | TU | WE | TH | FR | SA

Month/Week: ....

FOOD, NUTRITION & MEDS

	Carbs	Sugars	Fiber	Protein	Fat	Calories
BREAKFAST Time: .... Meds/Insulin						
Breakfast Total						
SNACK 1 Time: .... Meds/Insulin						
Snack 1 Total						
LUNCH Time: .... Meds/Insulin						
Lunch Total						
SNACK 2 Time: .... Meds/Insulin						
Snack 2 Total						
DINNER Time: .... Meds/Insulin						
Dinner Total						
Total Nutrition for the Day						

Water Consumption ⬜⬜⬜⬜⬜⬜⬜⬜⬜

BLOOD SUGAR LOG

	Blood Sugar Level	
	Before	After
WAKING-UP Time:	Sleep Hrs:	
	Fast. Hrs :	
BREAKFAST		
SNACK 1		
LUNCH		
SNACK 2		
DINNER		
BEDTIME	Go to Sleep Time:	

BLOOD PRESSURE & WEIGHT

Time	SYS/DIA	Pulse

WEIGHT: ....

NOTES/SCHEDULE

7 am
8 am
9 am
10 am
11 am
12 pm
1 pm
2 pm
3 pm
4 pm
5 pm
6 pm
7 pm
8 pm

EXERCISE & ACTIVITY LOG

	Time/Duration	Intensity/Calories

DATE: | SU | MO | TU | WE | TH | FR | SA

Month/ Week:

FOOD, NUTRITION & MEDS

	Carbs	Sugars	Fiber	Protein	Fat	Calories

BREAKFAST Time: .... Meds/ Insulin

Breakfast Total

SNACK 1 Time: .... Meds/ Insulin

Snack 1 Total

LUNCH Time: .... Meds/ Insulin

Lunch Total

SNACK 2 Time: .... Meds/ Insulin

Snack 2 Total

DINNER Time: .... Meds/ Insulin

Dinner Total

Total Nutrition for the Day

Water Consumption 🥛🥛🥛🥛🥛🥛🥛🥛🥛

EXERCISE & ACTIVITY LOG

Time/Duration   Intensity/Calories

BLOOD SUGAR LOG

	Blood Sugar Level	
	Before	After
WAKING-UP Time:	Sleep Hrs: .... Fast. Hrs :	
BREAKFAST		
SNACK 1		
LUNCH		
SNACK 2		
DINNER		
BEDTIME	Go to Sleep Time:	

BLOOD PRESSURE & WEIGHT

Time	SYS/DIA	Pulse

WEIGHT:

NOTES/SCHEDULE

7 am
8 am
9 am
10 am
11 am
12 pm
1 pm
2 pm
3 pm
4 pm
5 pm
6 pm
7 pm
8 pm

DATE:	SU	MO	TU	WE	TH	FR	SA	Month/ Week:

FOOD, NUTRITION & MEDS

	Carbs	Sugars	Fiber	Protein	Fat	Calories
BREAKFAST Time:	Meds/ Insulin					
Breakfast Total						
SNACK 1 Time:	Meds/ Insulin					
Snack 1 Total						
LUNCH Time:	Meds/ Insulin					
Lunch Total						
SNACK 2 Time:	Meds/ Insulin					
Snack 2 Total						
DINNER Time:	Meds/ Insulin					
Dinner Total						
Total Nutrition for the Day						

Water Consumption

EXERCISE & ACTIVITY LOG

	Time/Duration	Intensity/Calories

BLOOD SUGAR LOG

	Blood Sugar Level	
	Before	After
WAKING-UP Time:	Sleep Hrs: Fast. Hrs :	
BREAKFAST		
SNACK 1		
LUNCH		
SNACK 2		
DINNER		
BEDTIME	Go to Sleep Time:	

BLOOD PRESSURE & WEIGHT

Time	SYS/DIA	Pulse

WEIGHT:

NOTES/SCHEDULE

7 am
8 am
9 am
10 am
11 am
12 pm
1 pm
2 pm
3 pm
4 pm
5 pm
6 pm
7 pm
8 pm

DATE:		SU	MO	TU	WE	TH	FR	SA		Month/ Week:

FOOD, NUTRITION & MEDS

	Carbs	Sugars	Fiber	Protein	Fat	Calories
BREAKFAST Time: .... Meds/Insulin						
Breakfast Total						
SNACK 1 Time: .... Meds/Insulin						
Snack 1 Total						
LUNCH Time: .... Meds/Insulin						
Lunch Total						
SNACK 2 Time: .... Meds/Insulin						
Snack 2 Total						
DINNER Time: .... Meds/Insulin						
Dinner Total						
Total Nutrition for the Day						

Water Consumption ⬜⬜⬜⬜⬜⬜⬜⬜⬜ ....

EXERCISE & ACTIVITY LOG

	Time/Duration	Intensity/Calories

BLOOD SUGAR LOG

	Blood Sugar Level	
	Before	After
WAKING-UP Time:	Sleep Hrs: Fast. Hrs :	
BREAKFAST		
SNACK 1		
LUNCH		
SNACK 2		
DINNER		
BEDTIME	Go to Sleep Time:	

BLOOD PRESSURE & WEIGHT

Time	SYS/DIA	Pulse

WEIGHT: ....

NOTES/SCHEDULE

7 am
8 am
9 am
10 am
11 am
12 pm
1 pm
2 pm
3 pm
4 pm
5 pm
6 pm
7 pm
8 pm

FOOD, NUTRITION & MEDS

	Carbs	Sugars	Fiber	Protein	Fat	Calories
BREAKFAST Time: .... Meds/Insulin						
Breakfast Total						
SNACK 1 Time: .... Meds/Insulin						
Snack 1 Total						
LUNCH Time: .... Meds/Insulin						
Lunch Total						
SNACK 2 Time: .... Meds/Insulin						
Snack 2 Total						
DINNER Time: .... Meds/Insulin						
Dinner Total						
Total Nutrition for the Day						

Water Consumption ▢ ▢ ▢ ▢ ▢ ▢ ▢ ▢ ▢

EXERCISE & ACTIVITY LOG

	Time/Duration	Intensity/Calories

BLOOD SUGAR LOG

	Blood Sugar Level	
	Before	After
WAKING-UP Time:	Sleep Hrs: ...... Fast. Hrs :	
BREAKFAST		
SNACK 1		
LUNCH		
SNACK 2		
DINNER		
BEDTIME	Go to Sleep Time:	

BLOOD PRESSURE & WEIGHT

Time	SYS/DIA	Pulse

WEIGHT:

NOTES/SCHEDULE

7 am
8 am
9 am
10 am
11 am
12 pm
1 pm
2 pm
3 pm
4 pm
5 pm
6 pm
7 pm
8 pm

DATE:	SU	MO	TU	WE	TH	FR	SA	Month/ Week:

FOOD, NUTRITION & MEDS

	Carbs	Sugars	Fiber	Protein	Fat	Calories
BREAKFAST Time: _____ Meds/Insulin _____						
Breakfast Total						
SNACK 1 Time: _____ Meds/Insulin _____						
Snack 1 Total						
LUNCH Time: _____ Meds/Insulin _____						
Lunch Total						
SNACK 2 Time: _____ Meds/Insulin _____						
Snack 2 Total						
DINNER Time: _____ Meds/Insulin _____						
Dinner Total						
Total Nutrition for the Day						

Water Consumption ☐ ☐ ☐ ☐ ☐ ☐ ☐ ☐ ☐

EXERCISE & ACTIVITY LOG

	Time/Duration	Intensity/Calories

BLOOD SUGAR LOG

	Blood Sugar Level	
	Before	After
WAKING-UP Time:	Sleep Hrs: _____ Fast. Hrs : _____	
BREAKFAST		
SNACK 1		
LUNCH		
SNACK 2		
DINNER		
BEDTIME	Go to Sleep Time:	

BLOOD PRESSURE & WEIGHT

Time	SYS/DIA	Pulse
WEIGHT:		

NOTES/SCHEDULE

7 am	
8 am	
9 am	
10 am	
11 am	
12 pm	
1 pm	
2 pm	
3 pm	
4 pm	
5 pm	
6 pm	
7 pm	
8 pm	

FOOD, NUTRITION & MEDS

	Carbs	Sugars	Fiber	Protein	Fat	Calories
BREAKFAST Time: — Meds/Insulin						
Breakfast Total						
SNACK 1 Time: — Meds/Insulin						
Snack 1 Total						
LUNCH Time: — Meds/Insulin						
Lunch Total						
SNACK 2 Time: — Meds/Insulin						
Snack 2 Total						
DINNER Time: — Meds/Insulin						
Dinner Total						
Total Nutrition for the Day						

Water Consumption

EXERCISE & ACTIVITY LOG

	Time/Duration	Intensity/Calories

BLOOD SUGAR LOG

	Blood Sugar Level	
	Before	After
WAKING-UP Time:	Sleep Hrs: / Fast. Hrs :	
BREAKFAST		
SNACK 1		
LUNCH		
SNACK 2		
DINNER		
BEDTIME	Go to Sleep Time:	

BLOOD PRESSURE & WEIGHT

Time	SYS/DIA	Pulse

WEIGHT:

NOTES/SCHEDULE

7 am
8 am
9 am
10 am
11 am
12 pm
1 pm
2 pm
3 pm
4 pm
5 pm
6 pm
7 pm
8 pm

DATE:		SU	MO	TU	WE	TH	FR	SA	Month/ Week:

FOOD, NUTRITION & MEDS

	Carbs	Sugars	Fiber	Protein	Fat	Calories
BREAKFAST Time: .... Meds/ Insulin						
Breakfast Total						
SNACK 1 Time: .... Meds/ Insulin						
Snack 1 Total						
LUNCH Time: .... Meds/ Insulin						
Lunch Total						
SNACK 2 Time: .... Meds/ Insulin						
Snack 2 Total						
DINNER Time: .... Meds/ Insulin						
Dinner Total						
Total Nutrition for the Day						

Water Consumption ☐ ☐ ☐ ☐ ☐ ☐ ☐ ☐ ☐

EXERCISE & ACTIVITY LOG

	Time/Duration	Intensity/Calories

BLOOD SUGAR LOG

	Blood Sugar Level	
	Before	After
WAKING-UP Time:	Sleep Hrs: Fast. Hrs :	
BREAKFAST		
SNACK 1		
LUNCH		
SNACK 2		
DINNER		
BEDTIME	Go to Sleep Time:	

BLOOD PRESSURE & WEIGHT

Time	SYS/DIA	Pulse
WEIGHT:		

NOTES/SCHEDULE

7 am
8 am
9 am
10 am
11 am
12 pm
1 pm
2 pm
3 pm
4 pm
5 pm
6 pm
7 pm
8 pm

DATE: .... | SU | MO | TU | WE | TH | FR | SA |

Month/ Week: ....

FOOD, NUTRITION & MEDS

	Carbs	Sugars	Fiber	Protein	Fat	Calories

BREAKFAST Time: .... Meds/ Insulin ....

Breakfast Total						

SNACK 1 Time: .... Meds/ Insulin ....

Snack 1 Total						

LUNCH Time: .... Meds/ Insulin ....

Lunch Total						

SNACK 2 Time: .... Meds/ Insulin ....

Snack 2 Total						

DINNER Time: .... Meds/ Insulin ....

Dinner Total						
Total Nutrition for the Day						

Water Consumption ⬜⬜⬜⬜⬜⬜⬜⬜⬜

EXERCISE & ACTIVITY LOG

	Time/Duration	Intensity/Calories

BLOOD SUGAR LOG

	Blood Sugar Level	
	Before	After
WAKING-UP Time:	Sleep Hrs: Fast. Hrs :	
BREAKFAST		
SNACK 1		
LUNCH		
SNACK 2		
DINNER		
BEDTIME	Go to Sleep Time:	

BLOOD PRESSURE & WEIGHT

Time	SYS/DIA	Pulse

WEIGHT: ....

NOTES/SCHEDULE

7 am
8 am
9 am
10 am
11 am
12 pm
1 pm
2 pm
3 pm
4 pm
5 pm
6 pm
7 pm
8 pm

DATE:		SU	MO	TU	WE	TH	FR	SA		Month/ Week:

FOOD, NUTRITION & MEDS

	Carbs	Sugars	Fiber	Protein	Fat	Calories
BREAKFAST Time: .... Meds/Insulin						
Breakfast Total						
SNACK 1 Time: .... Meds/Insulin						
Snack 1 Total						
LUNCH Time: .... Meds/Insulin						
Lunch Total						
SNACK 2 Time: .... Meds/Insulin						
Snack 2 Total						
DINNER Time: .... Meds/Insulin						
Dinner Total						
Total Nutrition for the Day						

Water Consumption 🥛🥛🥛🥛🥛🥛🥛🥛🥛

EXERCISE & ACTIVITY LOG

	Time/Duration	Intensity/Calories

BLOOD SUGAR LOG

	Blood Sugar Level	
	Before	After
WAKING-UP Time:	Sleep Hrs: .... Fast. Hrs :	
BREAKFAST		
SNACK 1		
LUNCH		
SNACK 2		
DINNER		
BEDTIME	Go to Sleep Time:	

BLOOD PRESSURE & WEIGHT

Time	SYS/DIA	Pulse
WEIGHT:		

NOTES/SCHEDULE

7 am
8 am
9 am
10 am
11 am
12 pm
1 pm
2 pm
3 pm
4 pm
5 pm
6 pm
7 pm
8 pm

DATE:

SU	MO	TU	WE	TH	FR	SA

Month/
Week: ....

FOOD, NUTRITION & MEDS

	Carbs	Sugars	Fiber	Protein	Fat	Calories
BREAKFAST Time: .... Meds/Insulin						
Breakfast Total						
SNACK 1 Time: .... Meds/Insulin						
Snack 1 Total						
LUNCH Time: .... Meds/Insulin						
Lunch Total						
SNACK 2 Time: .... Meds/Insulin						
Snack 2 Total						
DINNER Time: .... Meds/Insulin						
Dinner Total						
Total Nutrition for the Day						

Water Consumption 🥛🥛🥛🥛🥛🥛🥛🥛🥛

EXERCISE & ACTIVITY LOG

	Time/Duration	Intensity/Calories

BLOOD SUGAR LOG

	Blood Sugar Level	
	Before	After
WAKING-UP Time:	Sleep Hrs: Fast. Hrs :	
BREAKFAST		
SNACK 1		
LUNCH		
SNACK 2		
DINNER		
BEDTIME	Go to Sleep Time:	

BLOOD PRESSURE & WEIGHT

Time	SYS/DIA	Pulse

WEIGHT:

NOTES/SCHEDULE

7 am
8 am
9 am
10 am
11 am
12 pm
1 pm
2 pm
3 pm
4 pm
5 pm
6 pm
7 pm
8 pm

DATE:	SU	MO	TU	WE	TH	FR	SA		Month/ Week:

FOOD, NUTRITION & MEDS

	Carbs	Sugars	Fiber	Protein	Fat	Calories
BREAKFAST Time:	Meds/ Insulin					
Breakfast Total						
SNACK 1 Time:	Meds/ Insulin					
Snack 1 Total						
LUNCH Time:	Meds/ Insulin					
Lunch Total						
SNACK 2 Time:	Meds/ Insulin					
Snack 2 Total						
DINNER Time:	Meds/ Insulin					
Dinner Total						
Total Nutrition for the Day						

Water Consumption

EXERCISE & ACTIVITY LOG

	Time/Duration	Intensity/Calories

BLOOD SUGAR LOG

	Blood Sugar Level	
	Before	After
WAKING-UP Time:	Sleep Hrs: Fast. Hrs :	
BREAKFAST		
SNACK 1		
LUNCH		
SNACK 2		
DINNER		
BEDTIME	Go to Sleep Time:	

BLOOD PRESSURE & WEIGHT

Time	SYS/DIA	Pulse
WEIGHT:		

NOTES/SCHEDULE

7 am
8 am
9 am
10 am
11 am
12 pm
1 pm
2 pm
3 pm
4 pm
5 pm
6 pm
7 pm
8 pm

DATE:	SU	MO	TU	WE	TH	FR	SA		Month/ Week:

FOOD, NUTRITION & MEDS

	Carbs	Sugars	Fiber	Protein	Fat	Calories
BREAKFAST Time:	Meds/ Insulin					
Breakfast Total						
SNACK 1 Time:	Meds/ Insulin					
Snack 1 Total						
LUNCH Time:	Meds/ Insulin					
Lunch Total						
SNACK 2 Time:	Meds/ Insulin					
Snack 2 Total						
DINNER Time:	Meds/ Insulin					
Dinner Total						
Total Nutrition for the Day						

Water Consumption ⬚⬚⬚⬚⬚⬚⬚⬚⬚

BLOOD SUGAR LOG

	Blood Sugar Level	
	Before	After
WAKING-UP Time:	Sleep Hrs: Fast. Hrs :	
BREAKFAST		
SNACK 1		
LUNCH		
SNACK 2		
DINNER		
BEDTIME	Go to Sleep Time:	

BLOOD PRESSURE & WEIGHT

Time	SYS/DIA	Pulse

WEIGHT:

NOTES/SCHEDULE

7 am
8 am
9 am
10 am
11 am
12 pm
1 pm
2 pm
3 pm
4 pm
5 pm
6 pm
7 pm
8 pm

EXERCISE & ACTIVITY LOG

	Time/Duration	Intensity/Calories

DATE:		SU	MO	TU	WE	TH	FR	SA	Month/ Week:

FOOD, NUTRITION & MEDS

	Carbs	Sugars	Fiber	Protein	Fat	Calories
BREAKFAST Time: .... Meds/Insulin						
Breakfast Total						
SNACK 1 Time: .... Meds/Insulin						
Snack 1 Total						
LUNCH Time: .... Meds/Insulin						
Lunch Total						
SNACK 2 Time: .... Meds/Insulin						
Snack 2 Total						
DINNER Time: .... Meds/Insulin						
Dinner Total						
Total Nutrition for the Day						

Water Consumption ▭ ▭ ▭ ▭ ▭ ▭ ▭ ▭ ▭ ▭ ....

EXERCISE & ACTIVITY LOG

	Time/Duration	Intensity/Calories

BLOOD SUGAR LOG

	Blood Sugar Level	
	Before	After
WAKING-UP Time:	Sleep Hrs: .... Fast. Hrs :	
BREAKFAST		
SNACK 1		
LUNCH		
SNACK 2		
DINNER		
BEDTIME	Go to Sleep Time:	

BLOOD PRESSURE & WEIGHT

Time	SYS/DIA	Pulse
WEIGHT:		

NOTES/SCHEDULE

7 am
8 am
9 am
10 am
11 am
12 pm
1 pm
2 pm
3 pm
4 pm
5 pm
6 pm
7 pm
8 pm

DATE:	SU	MO	TU	WE	TH	FR	SA	Month/Week:

FOOD, NUTRITION & MEDS

	Carbs	Sugars	Fiber	Protein	Fat	Calories
BREAKFAST Time: _____ Meds/Insulin _____						
Breakfast Total						
SNACK 1 Time: _____ Meds/Insulin _____						
Snack 1 Total						
LUNCH Time: _____ Meds/Insulin _____						
Lunch Total						
SNACK 2 Time: _____ Meds/Insulin _____						
Snack 2 Total						
DINNER Time: _____ Meds/Insulin _____						
Dinner Total						
Total Nutrition for the Day						

Water Consumption ⊔ ⊔ ⊔ ⊔ ⊔ ⊔ ⊔ ⊔ ⊔

BLOOD SUGAR LOG

	Blood Sugar Level	
	Before	After
WAKING-UP Time:	Sleep Hrs: Fast. Hrs :	
BREAKFAST		
SNACK 1		
LUNCH		
SNACK 2		
DINNER		
BEDTIME	Go to Sleep Time:	

BLOOD PRESSURE & WEIGHT

Time	SYS/DIA	Pulse

WEIGHT:

NOTES/SCHEDULE

7 am
8 am
9 am
10 am
11 am
12 pm
1 pm
2 pm
3 pm
4 pm
5 pm
6 pm
7 pm
8 pm

EXERCISE & ACTIVITY LOG

	Time/Duration	Intensity/Calories

DATE:	SU	MO	TU	WE	TH	FR	SA	Month/ Week:

FOOD, NUTRITION & MEDS

	Carbs	Sugars	Fiber	Protein	Fat	Calories
BREAKFAST Time: Meds/Insulin						
Breakfast Total						
SNACK 1 Time: Meds/Insulin						
Snack 1 Total						
LUNCH Time: Meds/Insulin						
Lunch Total						
SNACK 2 Time: Meds/Insulin						
Snack 2 Total						
DINNER Time: Meds/Insulin						
Dinner Total						
Total Nutrition for the Day						

Water Consumption ⬜⬜⬜⬜⬜⬜⬜⬜⬜⬜

EXERCISE & ACTIVITY LOG

	Time/Duration	Intensity/Calories

BLOOD SUGAR LOG

	Blood Sugar Level	
	Before	After
WAKING-UP Time:	Sleep Hrs: Fast. Hrs :	
BREAKFAST		
SNACK 1		
LUNCH		
SNACK 2		
DINNER		
BEDTIME	Go to Sleep Time:	

BLOOD PRESSURE & WEIGHT

Time	SYS/DIA	Pulse

WEIGHT:

NOTES/SCHEDULE

7 am
8 am
9 am
10 am
11 am
12 pm
1 pm
2 pm
3 pm
4 pm
5 pm
6 pm
7 pm
8 pm

Month/Week: ....

FOOD, NUTRITION & MEDS

	Carbs	Sugars	Fiber	Protein	Fat	Calories
BREAKFAST Time: .... Meds/Insulin						
Breakfast Total						
SNACK 1 Time: .... Meds/Insulin						
Snack 1 Total						
LUNCH Time: .... Meds/Insulin						
Lunch Total						
SNACK 2 Time: .... Meds/Insulin						
Snack 2 Total						
DINNER Time: .... Meds/Insulin						
Dinner Total						
Total Nutrition for the Day						

Water Consumption ▢ ▢ ▢ ▢ ▢ ▢ ▢ ▢ ▢

EXERCISE & ACTIVITY LOG

	Time/Duration	Intensity/Calories

BLOOD SUGAR LOG

	Blood Sugar Level	
	Before	After
WAKING-UP Time:	Sleep Hrs: Fast. Hrs :	
BREAKFAST		
SNACK 1		
LUNCH		
SNACK 2		
DINNER		
BEDTIME	Go to Sleep Time:	

BLOOD PRESSURE & WEIGHT

Time	SYS/DIA	Pulse

WEIGHT: ....

NOTES/SCHEDULE

7 am
8 am
9 am
10 am
11 am
12 pm
1 pm
2 pm
3 pm
4 pm
5 pm
6 pm
7 pm
8 pm

| DATE: | | SU | MO | TU | WE | TH | FR | SA | Month/ Week: |

FOOD, NUTRITION & MEDS

	Carbs	Sugars	Fiber	Protein	Fat	Calories
BREAKFAST Time: _____ Meds/ Insulin						
Breakfast Total						
SNACK 1 Time: _____ Meds/ Insulin						
Snack 1 Total						
LUNCH Time: _____ Meds/ Insulin						
Lunch Total						
SNACK 2 Time: _____ Meds/ Insulin						
Snack 2 Total						
DINNER Time: _____ Meds/ Insulin						
Dinner Total						
Total Nutrition for the Day						

Water Consumption ⬜⬜⬜⬜ ⬜⬜⬜⬜⬜

EXERCISE & ACTIVITY LOG

	Time/Duration	Intensity/Calories

BLOOD SUGAR LOG

	Blood Sugar Level	
	Before	After
WAKING-UP Time:	Sleep Hrs: Fast. Hrs :	
BREAKFAST		
SNACK 1		
LUNCH		
SNACK 2		
DINNER		
BEDTIME	Go to Sleep Time:	

BLOOD PRESSURE & WEIGHT

Time	SYS/DIA	Pulse
WEIGHT:		

NOTES/SCHEDULE

7 am
8 am
9 am
10 am
11 am
12 pm
1 pm
2 pm
3 pm
4 pm
5 pm
6 pm
7 pm
8 pm

DATE: .... | SU | MO | TU | WE | TH | FR | SA | **Month/ Week:** ....

FOOD, NUTRITION & MEDS

	Carbs	Sugars	Fiber	Protein	Fat	Calories
BREAKFAST Time: .... Meds/Insulin						
Breakfast Total						
SNACK 1 Time: .... Meds/Insulin						
Snack 1 Total						
LUNCH Time: .... Meds/Insulin						
Lunch Total						
SNACK 2 Time: .... Meds/Insulin						
Snack 2 Total						
DINNER Time: .... Meds/Insulin						
Dinner Total						
Total Nutrition for the Day						

Water Consumption ☐ ☐ ☐ ☐ ☐ ☐ ☐ ☐ ☐

EXERCISE & ACTIVITY LOG

	Time/Duration	Intensity/Calories

BLOOD SUGAR LOG

	Blood Sugar Level	
	Before	After
WAKING-UP Time:	Sleep Hrs: Fast. Hrs :	
BREAKFAST		
SNACK 1		
LUNCH		
SNACK 2		
DINNER		
BEDTIME	Go to Sleep Time:	

BLOOD PRESSURE & WEIGHT

Time	SYS/DIA	Pulse

WEIGHT:

NOTES/SCHEDULE

7 am
8 am
9 am
10 am
11 am
12 pm
1 pm
2 pm
3 pm
4 pm
5 pm
6 pm
7 pm
8 pm

| DATE: | | SU | MO | TU | WE | TH | FR | SA | Month/ Week: |

FOOD, NUTRITION & MEDS

	Carbs	Sugars	Fiber	Protein	Fat	Calories
BREAKFAST Time:	Meds/ Insulin					
Breakfast Total						
SNACK 1 Time:	Meds/ Insulin					
Snack 1 Total						
LUNCH Time:	Meds/ Insulin					
Lunch Total						
SNACK 2 Time:	Meds/ Insulin					
Snack 2 Total						
DINNER Time:	Meds/ Insulin					
Dinner Total						
Total Nutrition for the Day						

Water Consumption 🥛🥛🥛🥛🥛🥛🥛🥛🥛🥛 ....

EXERCISE & ACTIVITY LOG

	Time/Duration	Intensity/Calories

BLOOD SUGAR LOG

	Blood Sugar Level	
	Before	After
WAKING-UP Time:	Sleep Hrs: Fast. Hrs :	
BREAKFAST		
SNACK 1		
LUNCH		
SNACK 2		
DINNER		
BEDTIME	Go to Sleep Time:	

BLOOD PRESSURE & WEIGHT

Time	SYS/DIA	Pulse
WEIGHT:		

NOTES/SCHEDULE

7 am
8 am
9 am
10 am
11 am
12 pm
1 pm
2 pm
3 pm
4 pm
5 pm
6 pm
7 pm
8 pm

DATE: .... | SU | MO | TU | WE | TH | FR | SA | **Month/ Week:** ....

FOOD, NUTRITION & MEDS

	Carbs	Sugars	Fiber	Protein	Fat	Calories
BREAKFAST Time: .... Meds/ Insulin						
Breakfast Total						
SNACK 1 Time: .... Meds/ Insulin						
Snack 1 Total						
LUNCH Time: .... Meds/ Insulin						
Lunch Total						
SNACK 2 Time: .... Meds/ Insulin						
Snack 2 Total						
DINNER Time: .... Meds/ Insulin						
Dinner Total						
Total Nutrition for the Day						

Water Consumption ☐ ☐ ☐ ☐ ☐ ☐ ☐ ☐

EXERCISE & ACTIVITY LOG

	Time/Duration	Intensity/Calories

BLOOD SUGAR LOG

	Blood Sugar Level	
	Before	After
WAKING-UP Time:	Sleep Hrs: .... Fast. Hrs:	
BREAKFAST		
SNACK 1		
LUNCH		
SNACK 2		
DINNER		
BEDTIME	Go to Sleep Time:	

BLOOD PRESSURE & WEIGHT

Time	SYS/DIA	Pulse

WEIGHT:

NOTES/SCHEDULE

7 am
8 am
9 am
10 am
11 am
12 pm
1 pm
2 pm
3 pm
4 pm
5 pm
6 pm
7 pm
8 pm

DATE: .... | SU | MO | TU | WE | TH | FR | SA

Month/ Week: ....

FOOD, NUTRITION & MEDS

	Carbs	Sugars	Fiber	Protein	Fat	Calories

BREAKFAST Time: .... Meds/ Insulin

Breakfast Total

SNACK 1 Time: .... Meds/ Insulin

Snack 1 Total

LUNCH Time: .... Meds/ Insulin

Lunch Total

SNACK 2 Time: .... Meds/ Insulin

Snack 2 Total

DINNER Time: .... Meds/ Insulin

Dinner Total

Total Nutrition for the Day

Water Consumption ⊔ ⊔ ⊔ ⊔ ⊔ ⊔ ⊔ ⊔ ⊔ ⊔

EXERCISE & ACTIVITY LOG

Time/Duration | Intensity/Calories

BLOOD SUGAR LOG

	Blood Sugar Level	
	Before	After
WAKING-UP Time:	Sleep Hrs: Fast. Hrs :	
BREAKFAST		
SNACK 1		
LUNCH		
SNACK 2		
DINNER		
BEDTIME	Go to Sleep Time:	

BLOOD PRESSURE & WEIGHT

Time	SYS/DIA	Pulse

WEIGHT:

NOTES/SCHEDULE

7 am
8 am
9 am
10 am
11 am
12 pm
1 pm
2 pm
3 pm
4 pm
5 pm
6 pm
7 pm
8 pm

DATE:		SU	MO	TU	WE	TH	FR	SA	Month/ Week:

FOOD, NUTRITION & MEDS

	Carbs	Sugars	Fiber	Protein	Fat	Calories

BREAKFAST Time:
Meds/ Insulin

Breakfast Total

SNACK 1 Time:
Meds/ Insulin

Snack 1 Total

LUNCH Time:
Meds/ Insulin

Lunch Total

SNACK 2 Time:
Meds/ Insulin

Snack 2 Total

DINNER Time:
Meds/ Insulin

Dinner Total

Total Nutrition for the Day

Water Consumption

EXERCISE & ACTIVITY LOG

	Time/Duration	Intensity/Calories

BLOOD SUGAR LOG

	Blood Sugar Level	
	Before	After
WAKING-UP Time:	Sleep Hrs: Fast. Hrs :	
BREAKFAST		
SNACK 1		
LUNCH		
SNACK 2		
DINNER		
BEDTIME	Go to Sleep Time:	

BLOOD PRESSURE & WEIGHT

Time	SYS/DIA	Pulse

WEIGHT:

NOTES/SCHEDULE

7 am
8 am
9 am
10 am
11 am
12 pm
1 pm
2 pm
3 pm
4 pm
5 pm
6 pm
7 pm
8 pm

FOOD, NUTRITION & MEDS

	Carbs	Sugars	Fiber	Protein	Fat	Calories
BREAKFAST Time: .... Meds/ Insulin						
Breakfast Total						
SNACK 1 Time: .... Meds/ Insulin						
Snack 1 Total						
LUNCH Time: .... Meds/ Insulin						
Lunch Total						
SNACK 2 Time: .... Meds/ Insulin						
Snack 2 Total						
DINNER Time: .... Meds/ Insulin						
Dinner Total						
Total Nutrition for the Day						

Water Consumption ☐ ☐ ☐ ☐ ☐ ☐ ☐ ☐ ☐ ☐ ....

EXERCISE & ACTIVITY LOG

	Time/Duration	Intensity/Calories
....		
....		
....		
....		
....		

BLOOD SUGAR LOG

	Blood Sugar Level	
	Before	After
WAKING-UP Time:	Sleep Hrs: Fast. Hrs :	
BREAKFAST		
SNACK 1		
LUNCH		
SNACK 2		
DINNER		
BEDTIME	Go to Sleep Time:	

BLOOD PRESSURE & WEIGHT

Time	SYS/DIA	Pulse

WEIGHT: ....

NOTES/SCHEDULE

7 am ....
8 am ....
9 am ....
10 am ....
11 am ....
12 pm ....
1 pm ....
2 pm ....
3 pm ....
4 pm ....
5 pm ....
6 pm ....
7 pm ....
8 pm ....

DATE: .... | SU | MO | TU | WE | TH | FR | SA | Month/Week: ....

FOOD, NUTRITION & MEDS

	Carbs	Sugars	Fiber	Protein	Fat	Calories
BREAKFAST Time: .... Meds/Insulin						
Breakfast Total						
SNACK 1 Time: .... Meds/Insulin						
Snack 1 Total						
LUNCH Time: .... Meds/Insulin						
Lunch Total						
SNACK 2 Time: .... Meds/Insulin						
Snack 2 Total						
DINNER Time: .... Meds/Insulin						
Dinner Total						
Total Nutrition for the Day						

Water Consumption ▢ ▢ ▢ ▢ ▢ ▢ ▢ ▢ ▢

EXERCISE & ACTIVITY LOG

	Time/Duration	Intensity/Calories

BLOOD SUGAR LOG

	Blood Sugar Level	
	Before	After
WAKING-UP Time:	Sleep Hrs: Fast. Hrs :	
BREAKFAST		
SNACK 1		
LUNCH		
SNACK 2		
DINNER		
BEDTIME	Go to Sleep Time:	

BLOOD PRESSURE & WEIGHT

Time	SYS/DIA	Pulse

WEIGHT:

NOTES/SCHEDULE

7 am
8 am
9 am
10 am
11 am
12 pm
1 pm
2 pm
3 pm
4 pm
5 pm
6 pm
7 pm
8 pm

DATE: | SU | MO | TU | WE | TH | FR | SA | **Month/ Week:**

FOOD, NUTRITION & MEDS

	Carbs	Sugars	Fiber	Protein	Fat	Calories

BREAKFAST Time: .... Meds/ Insulin ....

Breakfast Total						

SNACK 1 Time: .... Meds/ Insulin ....

Snack 1 Total						

LUNCH Time: .... Meds/ Insulin ....

Lunch Total						

SNACK 2 Time: .... Meds/ Insulin ....

Snack 2 Total						

DINNER Time: .... Meds/ Insulin ....

Dinner Total						
Total Nutrition for the Day						

Water Consumption 🥛🥛🥛🥛🥛🥛🥛🥛🥛🥛

EXERCISE & ACTIVITY LOG

	Time/Duration	Intensity/Calories

BLOOD SUGAR LOG

	Blood Sugar Level	
	Before	After
WAKING-UP Time:	Sleep Hrs: Fast. Hrs :	
BREAKFAST		
SNACK 1		
LUNCH		
SNACK 2		
DINNER		
BEDTIME	Go to Sleep Time:	

BLOOD PRESSURE & WEIGHT

Time	SYS/DIA	Pulse
WEIGHT:		

NOTES/SCHEDULE

7 am
8 am
9 am
10 am
11 am
12 pm
1 pm
2 pm
3 pm
4 pm
5 pm
6 pm
7 pm
8 pm

DATE: | SU | MO | TU | WE | TH | FR | SA | **Month/ Week:**

FOOD, NUTRITION & MEDS

	Carbs	Sugars	Fiber	Protein	Fat	Calories

BREAKFAST   Time: Meds/Insulin

Breakfast Total

SNACK 1   Time: Meds/Insulin

Snack 1 Total

LUNCH   Time: Meds/Insulin

Lunch Total

SNACK 2   Time: Meds/Insulin

Snack 2 Total

DINNER   Time: Meds/Insulin

Dinner Total

Total Nutrition for the Day

Water Consumption

EXERCISE & ACTIVITY LOG

	Time/Duration	Intensity/Calories

BLOOD SUGAR LOG

	Blood Sugar Level	
	Before	After
WAKING-UP Time:	Sleep Hrs: Fast. Hrs :	
BREAKFAST		
SNACK 1		
LUNCH		
SNACK 2		
DINNER		
BEDTIME	Go to Sleep Time:	

BLOOD PRESSURE & WEIGHT

Time	SYS/DIA	Pulse

WEIGHT:

NOTES/SCHEDULE

7 am
8 am
9 am
10 am
11 am
12 pm
1 pm
2 pm
3 pm
4 pm
5 pm
6 pm
7 pm
8 pm

DATE: | SU | MO | TU | WE | TH | FR | SA   **Month/Week:**

FOOD, NUTRITION & MEDS

	Carbs	Sugars	Fiber	Protein	Fat	Calories
BREAKFAST Time: .... Meds/Insulin						
Breakfast Total						
SNACK 1 Time: .... Meds/Insulin						
Snack 1 Total						
LUNCH Time: .... Meds/Insulin						
Lunch Total						
SNACK 2 Time: .... Meds/Insulin						
Snack 2 Total						
DINNER Time: .... Meds/Insulin						
Dinner Total						
Total Nutrition for the Day						

Water Consumption ☐ ☐ ☐ ☐ ☐ ☐ ☐ ☐ ☐ ☐ ....

EXERCISE & ACTIVITY LOG

Time/Duration   Intensity/Calories

BLOOD SUGAR LOG

	Blood Sugar Level	
	Before	After
WAKING-UP Time:	Sleep Hrs: .... Fast. Hrs :	
BREAKFAST		
SNACK 1		
LUNCH		
SNACK 2		
DINNER		
BEDTIME	Go to Sleep Time:	

BLOOD PRESSURE & WEIGHT

Time	SYS/DIA	Pulse

WEIGHT:

NOTES/SCHEDULE

7 am
8 am
9 am
10 am
11 am
12 pm
1 pm
2 pm
3 pm
4 pm
5 pm
6 pm
7 pm
8 pm

DATE: .... | SU | MO | TU | WE | TH | FR | SA | **Month/ Week:** ....

FOOD, NUTRITION & MEDS

	Carbs	Sugars	Fiber	Protein	Fat	Calories
BREAKFAST Time: .... Meds/Insulin						
Breakfast Total						
SNACK 1 Time: .... Meds/Insulin						
Snack 1 Total						
LUNCH Time: .... Meds/Insulin						
Lunch Total						
SNACK 2 Time: .... Meds/Insulin						
Snack 2 Total						
DINNER Time: .... Meds/Insulin						
Dinner Total						
Total Nutrition for the Day						

Water Consumption ⬜ ⬜ ⬜ ⬜ ⬜ ⬜ ⬜ ⬜ ⬜

EXERCISE & ACTIVITY LOG

	Time/Duration	Intensity/Calories

BLOOD SUGAR LOG

	Blood Sugar Level	
	Before	After
WAKING-UP Time:	Sleep Hrs: Fast. Hrs :	
BREAKFAST		
SNACK 1		
LUNCH		
SNACK 2		
DINNER		
BEDTIME	Go to Sleep Time:	

BLOOD PRESSURE & WEIGHT

Time	SYS/DIA	Pulse

WEIGHT:

NOTES/SCHEDULE

7 am
8 am
9 am
10 am
11 am
12 pm
1 pm
2 pm
3 pm
4 pm
5 pm
6 pm
7 pm
8 pm

DATE:	SU	MO	TU	WE	TH	FR	SA	Month/Week:

FOOD, NUTRITION & MEDS

	Carbs	Sugars	Fiber	Protein	Fat	Calories
BREAKFAST Time:	Meds/Insulin					
Breakfast Total						
SNACK 1 Time:	Meds/Insulin					
Snack 1 Total						
LUNCH Time:	Meds/Insulin					
Lunch Total						
SNACK 2 Time:	Meds/Insulin					
Snack 2 Total						
DINNER Time:	Meds/Insulin					
Dinner Total						
Total Nutrition for the Day						

Water Consumption ⬜⬜⬜⬜⬜⬜⬜⬜⬜⬜

EXERCISE & ACTIVITY LOG

	Time/Duration	Intensity/Calories

BLOOD SUGAR LOG

	Blood Sugar Level	
	Before	After
WAKING-UP Time:	Sleep Hrs: Fast. Hrs :	
BREAKFAST		
SNACK 1		
LUNCH		
SNACK 2		
DINNER		
BEDTIME	Go to Sleep Time:	

BLOOD PRESSURE & WEIGHT

Time	SYS/DIA	Pulse

WEIGHT:

NOTES/SCHEDULE

7 am
8 am
9 am
10 am
11 am
12 pm
1 pm
2 pm
3 pm
4 pm
5 pm
6 pm
7 pm
8 pm

DATE: | SU | MO | TU | WE | TH | FR | SA | **Month/ Week:**

FOOD, NUTRITION & MEDS

	Carbs	Sugars	Fiber	Protein	Fat	Calories
BREAKFAST Time: — Meds/ Insulin						
Breakfast Total						
SNACK 1 Time: — Meds/ Insulin						
Snack 1 Total						
LUNCH Time: — Meds/ Insulin						
Lunch Total						
SNACK 2 Time: — Meds/ Insulin						
Snack 2 Total						
DINNER Time: — Meds/ Insulin						
Dinner Total						
Total Nutrition for the Day						

Water Consumption ⬜⬜⬜⬜⬜⬜⬜⬜⬜⬜

EXERCISE & ACTIVITY LOG

	Time/Duration	Intensity/Calories

BLOOD SUGAR LOG

	Blood Sugar Level	
	Before	After
WAKING-UP Time:	Sleep Hrs: Fast. Hrs :	
BREAKFAST		
SNACK 1		
LUNCH		
SNACK 2		
DINNER		
BEDTIME	Go to Sleep Time:	

BLOOD PRESSURE & WEIGHT

Time	SYS/DIA	Pulse

WEIGHT:

NOTES/SCHEDULE

7 am
8 am
9 am
10 am
11 am
12 pm
1 pm
2 pm
3 pm
4 pm
5 pm
6 pm
7 pm
8 pm

DATE:	SU	MO	TU	WE	TH	FR	SA	Month/ Week:

FOOD, NUTRITION & MEDS

	Carbs	Sugars	Fiber	Protein	Fat	Calories
BREAKFAST Time: .... Meds/Insulin						
Breakfast Total						
SNACK 1 Time: .... Meds/Insulin						
Snack 1 Total						
LUNCH Time: .... Meds/Insulin						
Lunch Total						
SNACK 2 Time: .... Meds/Insulin						
Snack 2 Total						
DINNER Time: .... Meds/Insulin						
Dinner Total						
Total Nutrition for the Day						

Water Consumption ▭ ▭ ▭ ▭ ▭ ▭ ▭ ▭ ....

BLOOD SUGAR LOG

	Blood Sugar Level	
	Before	After
WAKING-UP Time:	Sleep Hrs: .... Fast. Hrs :	
BREAKFAST		
SNACK 1		
LUNCH		
SNACK 2		
DINNER		
BEDTIME	Go to Sleep Time:	

BLOOD PRESSURE & WEIGHT

Time	SYS/DIA	Pulse
WEIGHT:		

NOTES/SCHEDULE

7 am
8 am
9 am
10 am
11 am
12 pm
1 pm
2 pm
3 pm
4 pm
5 pm
6 pm
7 pm
8 pm

EXERCISE & ACTIVITY LOG

	Time/Duration	Intensity/Calories

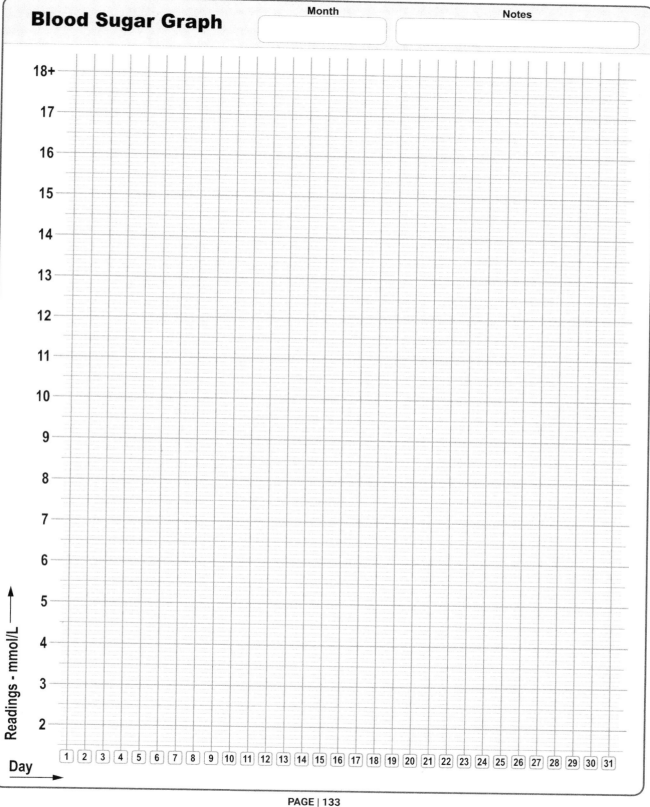

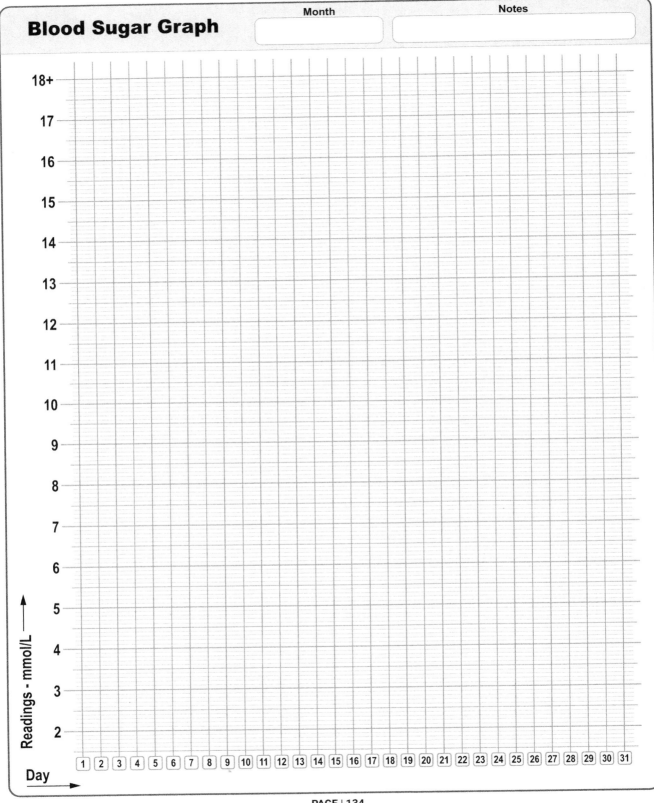

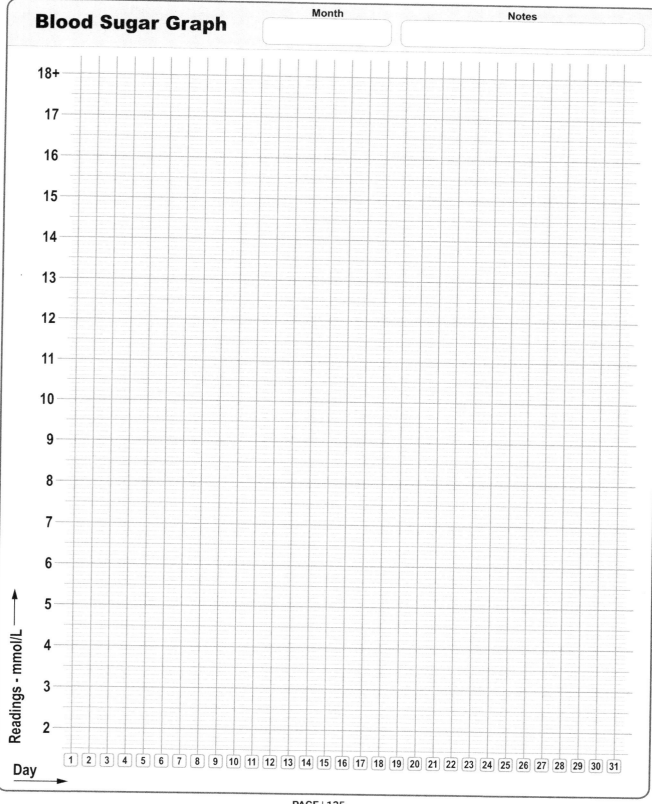

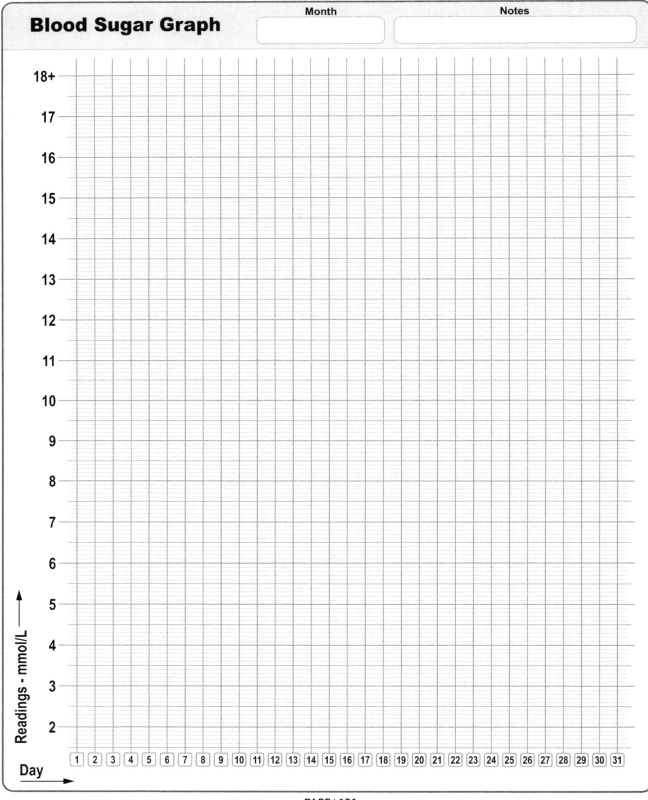

Medical Notes

Medical Notes

Medical Notes

Medical Notes